FALLING OUT OF NORMAL

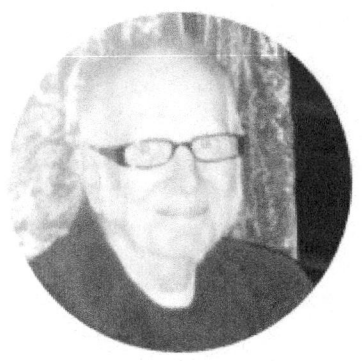

"How I Became Me."

———————

Allen L. Vance
established 1930

HOW I BECAME ME

FALLING OUT OF NORMAL
Copyright © 2018 by Allen L. Vance
Courtesy of publisher & bookmaker: (Daughter)
Janine Vance | Vance Twins
Cover design: Dustin Allen Vance (Grandson)

Photos of the house from zillow.com
Photos of Allen with glider, unknown.

All rights reserved. No part of this book may be reproduced or transmitted in any form or by any means without written permission from the author.

Contents

Wing-Nuts to Just Nuts 5
They Called Me Crazy 10
The 1930s: A Normal Nomad 19
The 1940s: A Typical Teenager 31
The 1950s: I was a Big Drip. You Dig? 49
The 1960s & 70s: Building a Life (and a House) 59
The 1980s: Falling Out of Normal 76
Retirement Years: Enjoying Isolation 85
Millennial Years: Making Peace with Not-Normal 95
Afterthoughts: On Why I Journaled 99

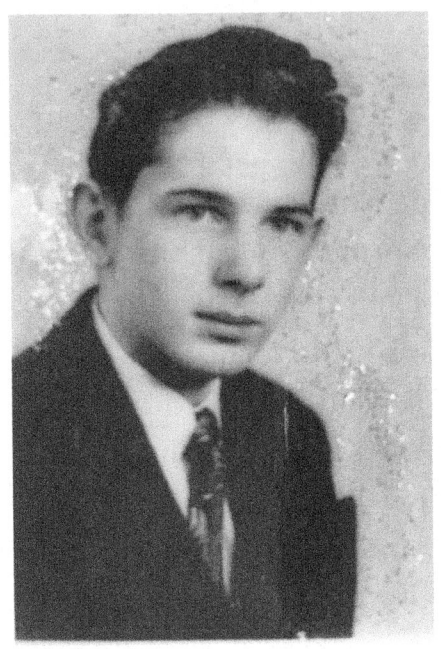

ALLEN LOUIS VANCE

"This writing will probably never become a published book, and that is okay with me. I wrote it as a personal record and for the fun of it. I think everyone should write a record of their life. No two lives are the same. It is amazing what one can learn from another's experience."
Allen

Wing-Nuts to Just Nuts

"The worst you can call me is normal."
-Allen

My history all started with my birth. I was born in 1930 and named Allen Louis Vance. I was born in a normal hospital in Portland, Oregon.

I didn't know how to talk yet, so I cried.

My life was normal at first. While I was a baby, a kid, a teenager, and then an adult, I was given the normal lie about everything. I never questioned what I was told. That included at home, in grade school, high school, at college, or by my friends; they all thought they knew how things worked and told me. I didn't have to think, just listen. It still amazes me that so many were so wrong about so much.

HOW I BECAME ME

I was even told that the Bible was true. I had read the King James Version (KJV) of the Bible, cover-to-cover, thirty-four times and believed it literally during the 1980s and through to the 90s.

My whole life changed one day in October of 1984. I forgot to install the two wing nuts that were meant to keep my cheap second-hand hang glider from folding during flight. You guessed what happened. Neither pilot (me) nor an experienced hang glider pilot had checked the wing to verify that it was ready for flight. It wasn't.

I was on Dog Mountain, intending to make my seventh "high altitude flight." A high altitude flight is one in which the altitude of the landing site is 1,000 feet lower or more in altitude than that of the take-off site. I had flown off Dog Mountain before and was very pleased with it as a take-off site.

It was early in the day, before the thermals. Thermals are masses of rising air caused by hot spots on the ground., like asphalt roads or plowed earth. Skilled pilots liked to fly in the late afternoon because they can soar like a bird in rising air from ground heat. My flight was to be a "Sled Ride." No thermals.

FALLING OUT OF NORMAL

Dog Mountain was covered with needle-type trees that grow like weeds. The trees probably saved my life. My falling speed was reduced by the tree I fell through, and contact with the ground could have done more damage than happened.

Without the wing-nuts, the glider wing folded per design, but I was in mid-flight at the time. I fell about fifty feet into a tree, fifty-five feet through the tree, and hit the ground hard enough to break the fiberglass helmet I was wearing. The fall usually killed the pilot, but my fall was severe enough to cause the redesign of future wings. (The wing-makers went to a pull cable design to rid the wing-nuts.)

The solution made a new wing slightly heavier and a little more costly and didn't solve the problem of no preflight inspection. Still, the experienced hang glider pilots were careful to check their own gliders before take-off. The subject of a preflight wing inspection never came up during class. I think the wing-nut design is better than a cable design, but I'm for a preflight inspection. They require a preflight inspection on all wings. No-one checked.

Post fall, I was told the pilots were instructed to put the wing-nuts in their mouth, and they would never forget to install them before a flight. I always wondered how many hang glider pilots forgot to put the wing-nuts in their mouth. If there was a fault, it was in preflight checking. In my case, there was none.

I got my first ride on a helicopter that day, but it was to a hospital. So came the end of hang gliding for me and the start of a new life. It was Oct 24, 1984, and I was still alive. I was like a new-born. Nothing I tried worked. I had to discover life all over.

While I was in the hospital, I had five surgeries. My left eye was out of place, and I developed a bone spur on my left elbow, which immobilized my left arm and kept it against my chest. I was unable to use my left arm at all. The operations finally got everything back where it belonged, and I was whole again.

I ended my job of thirty-two years with Boeing. I liked my job there, and for all the time I was with them, it never occurred to me that I was working on war machines. It was not until I became non-normal that I became aware that I was the foe.

We were always in a secret area, but I never thought to ask why.

After my hang-gliding fall, I was confined to a wheelchair for two years, but the parking is great. The United States Government gave me a flag to attach to the car's rearview mirror, allowing me to park in any un-used handicapped spot. These spots were usually right in front of the door to the place I was going. But all was not fun and games.

But I am getting ahead of myself. Let me tell you how I became non-normal.

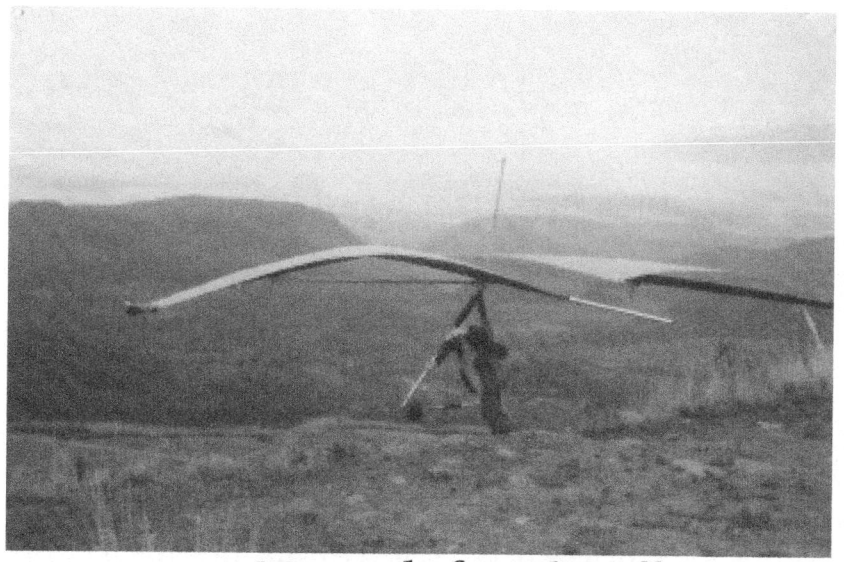

Me, ready for take-off.
(or not so ready)

HOW I BECAME ME

They Called Me Crazy

There were about 7.4 billion humans on earth in 2016, and the number is rising. Most of those people are normal. Let me define my difference between normal and non-normal: A normal reacts without thinking; a non-normal person thinks before acting. I should know. I've been both kinds of people.

Non-normals let the soul do that. They do not want to rock the boat, but they do not believe what the mass of normal people say they believe.

I have one edge that might drive you to say, "that's not fair," and you might be right. My edge is that my daughter and her sister are non-normal. It was not evident until my fall, than it became obvious. The way to be NON-NORMAL is to think. It is that simple. Most humans will live a whole lifetime and not think. They will memorize in school but not think about what they are memorizing. They will be graded on how well they remember, not what it said.

I have formed a mental picture about judgment. The mental picture is a horizontal line with LOVE on the left end and FEAR on the right end. When a person makes a choice, and they do that hundreds of times each day. They pick a spot on the line. God always knows what we are thinking and where we would place ourselves on the line. There is no need to wait for death for judgment. We do that every day.

We were made out of eternal stuff, and unless God is a liar, we are eternal. The body will die, but that is not us. My soul tells me I am on my 420th life. For example, the Bible tells of God as the creator, of, among other things, an adversary against Satan, who could win a war with God. My God is not that stupid. My God doesn't lose things like a War. My God does not need to "fight" a war. Only humans fight wars.

Some people have died and then been revived, yet there is no account from them of "Pearly Gates" or "Heaven" or "Hell." I have put the Bible down as being too hard to interpret. The Bible does not agree with people who have experienced an event. It is full of similarities, which makes it very hard to understand.

Death is only one of many places the Bible does not agree with experience. I, at least, find no value in studying the King James Version of the Bible.

People are told we only live one life, but that is not what my soul has conveyed to me. I align with the soul. Death is not the only place the Bible does not agree with. The KJV of the Bible makes no mention of reincarnation, even though the early Jewish Bible does. The reason given for this is that King David did not believe in reincarnation. My question is, How many other changes did King David make?

When I thought of myself as normal, I imagined that I was singular. Competition made sense to me. But no longer. It would be like the right hand competing with the left hand. My body does not work that way. The hands may look different, but they work together on all tasks. I believe people are like that. No person is alone; they are all part of oneness. Together, they are very powerful. Separate, they are weak.
That is very hard for me to realize, yet I see an example of that in my life.

I have a small black dog named Barklee. Supposedly, the dog is mine, but the whole family takes care of him. As long as the family and dog act the way they do, I have no concern.

My granddaughter Alli searched and found a small dog, because my big sixty-four-pound Chinese Shar-pei and bull-dog mix dog named Putt-Putt had caused me to fall, and he was powerful. The little black dog has slept with me for years. He has his own bed on my bed.
That may seem trivial to you, but it is only one of many changes in my life. Other changes include editing for free and yielding my place in line at the store as a customer who only wants to buy a few items.

NORMAL people spend most of their life trying to figure out their purpose for living, which is a big waste of time when God has already done that. Before God created humans, God mentally considered everything humans could do but could not come up with a method for experiencing it. The only thing that was important to God at the time was experiencing life. That is why I believe God to be the universal collective of all that is. All of us are included as part of the energetic field, which is God.

So God created the species called humans composed of the soul, which is part of God in my honest opinion. But you might never know this philosophy unless you meditated or talked with God (the universal oneness) or read *Conversations With God* (CWG). We are part of God, and our purpose is to simply be.

It doesn't matter to God if you are a doctor or a janitor. God's only concern is that you are alive. How are we like God? Simple, we can create. I know, I've done it! In my honest opinion, CWG is a must-read for anyone who cares what God is really like. I'm a big fan.

For a long time, normal people believed that the earth was flat and rode on the back of a giant turtle. I hope you are not one of them. We still call it sunrise; when the sun does not rise, the earth turns.

Humans make a big deal out of not changing history. Like we should keep old language when we know it's obsolete. For example, we know the sun doesn't rise or set, yet we still say "sunrise" and "sunset." Well, I think we should say something like "day start" and "night start."

There is one more step that most people take—at least I took—and that is always being busy. My adopted daughter avoided this situation by writing five books, babysitting her sister's child, and raising a family. She is always busy. Humans like that. They hate boredom. Boredom can lead to thoughts of suicide. This situation prompted me to write this book. My fall caused the loss of many time-fillers I had before my injury, such as water and snow skiing, car collecting, camping, working at Boeing, and driving. The irony is that we often do it to ourselves. But this is not Life's Purpose. This is just a purpose that we set for ourselves. It is really a self-conceived "time-filler" designed to offset boredom.

I ran the gamete of churches but ended with none. They were all teaching lies. I found more in CWG than in any church. The biggest lie is that we are born in sin. Another lie is that Jesus can save anyone but himself.

I like Neale Donald Walsh's saying, "I could be wrong . . . "Human beings are continually finding things they never understood before. It is with great conceit that many resist change as if we know it all. Humans tend to disregard anything that disagrees with any church. Maybe there is a church that has it right and I just have not found it yet. In the meantime, I'm a fan of the philosophy found in *Conversations with God.*

Another thought I found that was a significant change for me was that human beings never *own* anything. Things are only on loan to humans for a period. We are born with nothing, and we die the same way. Our children are the greatest example of that reality. Sired or adopted, they are only with us as babies, kids, teens, and part of their adult life, then they usually leave us to start their own families.

I should know because I raised four children. One sired and three adopted, and they all followed the formula.

Yes, there are "boomerang" kids that never leave the parents' home or leave it, then return to the parents at some later date, but the parents still die alone. The children may get so used to the lifestyle at the parent's home that the children hate to have less, but that is very unusual. Children are only loaned to parents to teach the kids how the world works. Once that is done, the parent's job is completed.

Another example of non-ownership is my house. I designed it myself, then built it with my own two hands. It had some features that most homes lack. For example, it was designed to house two families, one upstairs, the other downstairs. It had two separate front doors: one up, the other down. It had a huge septic tank that could easily handle two families. It had a full kitchen and refrigerator downstairs. In fact, during its construction, my wife, I, and two boys lived in the basement for a while. The fireplace could take a six-foot-long piece of wood to heat the basement if the oil furnace failed, but it never failed. The wooded lot could easily provide fuel. The fireplace had two flues, and the top was covered to prevent a down-draft. Steel tube beam tubes were used to prevent the house from being separated by earthquakes. The house had doors on opposite walls for exiting in case of fire. The house had an alarm system that would not keep one out but monitored the inside. The house was surrounded by a six-foot-high board fence, which kept people out and the two German Shepherd dogs inside. I always thought the house was mine, but all that changed with my injury. My wife divorced me, and the house got sold. It was no longer mine.

God can appear as anything God wants to be. For example, God can appear as a microbe, a river, a tree, a mountain, a planet, or a universe.

For years God has been called "he," but that is just one of the things God can appear as. God is surely not only a male. God is thought of by me as the ultimate shape-shifter. I believe God is some kind of energy that has no name, but we call it God.
There are a lot of things about God that I have yet to learn. For example: How can God not have a size or a beginning? These are just a couple of things I do not yet understand. The list goes on and on.

I can't imagine even a few things about mathematics, like infinity, but I use math anyway.

HOW I BECAME ME

The English language needs to add some words as a pronoun for God. In the meantime, I'll just use the word *God*.

It is not God's fault if our prayer of asking is not answered. We don't ask for what we have! A prayer of asking is an admission that we don't have whatever we ask for, or we would not ask for it. Only pray in gratitude.

Sometimes an answer takes time to be seen, but that doesn't mean it hasn't happened.

There is another thing about prayer that really scares me, I am not alone. What if my prayer is negated by another?

I try to keep my prayers only to influence myself in an effort to avoid someone else's prayer, which might negate my prayer.

(From the very beginning, they called me crazy. But, that's not my problem! If they call you crazy, you shouldn't care either. We just do things differently than everyone else.

~Allen)

The 1930s: A Normal Nomad

I was born in an Oregon hospital and spent the whole period in the city of Portland. I was too young to do anything, and I have no memory of this period of my life. Most of the time, I just grew and listened to my mother. My daughter recently bore a baby named Maya. My other daughter is now babysitting, Maya. She is a real-time task. At least we now have throw-away diapers. They were not available when I was an infant. The trouble is that our dump-sites are filling up with used diapers. Eventually, something will have to change.

My mother was employed by the Aladine company until I was born, then she became a stay-at-home mom. My father worked for Damascus Milk

Company, delivering special orders on a three-wheeled motorcycle.

Most of this writing is about my life when I got older. I didn't do much during this Life Phase.

Leader:
I was always a leader. I think I was born that way, but none of the kids I played with seemed to mind. I was always the proverbial nerd, but no one ever harassed or picked on me, and I never had to fight for any reason. It was not a conscious thing, this thing of being a leader, it was just a thing I was. Most of the time, I was ignored. Then a leader would be required, and that was my queue to step forward.

Portland, Oregon:
All the places I lived during this period of my life were in Portland, Oregon, which claimed to be the best place in the world. The weather was usually mild the year around, at least it was during my time there. It rained a lot but usually at night while I was asleep. That would not get me wet.

I only have one picture of my parents before they were married. They were standing in front of an old car, I don't even know what kind, it had a cloth top and seated six. They never told me when they were married or if they did, I don't remember.

FALLING OUT OF NORMAL

My father was drafted into the army during the first world war, but the war ended before he got shipped out. So he never saw combat. He was never even issued a rifle. Now you have all the introductory data, and I'll go on with my experiences.

Residence:
We lived in several places, but the one I remember best is the rented house in South Portland. It was in that house that I faithfully listened to the Lone Ranger on the radio. Television was not a household item yet, so I listened to the radio every evening. Since we had no television, the *Lone Ranger* and *Fibber Magee's Closet* were just pictured in my mind. It was also the period in my life where I sent for every decoder system offered. I could decode most secret messages, but I found that most of them were ads and not worth deciphering. The house was small, but then so was my family.

We lived near a store and walked to most places. I never saw my mother drive. I don't think she ever had a driver's license. Anyway, there was no extra car. My father always drove our only car, a fourth-one Oldsmobile.

It was in this house that I put a peanut in my nose and had to go to the doctor to get the peanut removed. The doctor's office was within walking distance, so we hoofed it. I learned one thing from that experience. How to get a peanut, or anything, out of the nose. With a finger, close-off the unaffected nose-port and blow out the other nose-port. It only took the doctor a few seconds to remove the peanut, and it did not require any special equipment. I could have avoided a doctor's visit.

Four More Residences:
For a while, I slept in an apartment over a grocery store on the *south-west* corner of Eleventh Avenue and Alberta Street located in north Portland. It was convenient for transportation, with streetcars running every ten minutes. You could board one, and it would take you right downtown for a dime. The thing I remember most about that place is the stairs up to my home. They were on the rear of the store, uncarpeted, wood stained dark, poorly lit, and seemed to go on forever.

From there, I moved two blocks north along Eleventh Avenue to Auntie Lee's house. She was my father's sister, and the house was the biggest in the whole neighborhood. It was two stories and had a full basement, with a concrete floor. The house was built in early 1911 and had more than four bedrooms. (Today, it supposedly has 11 bedrooms) Each downstairs bedroom was equipped with a sink. I never used the sink, but I had one, and it worked.

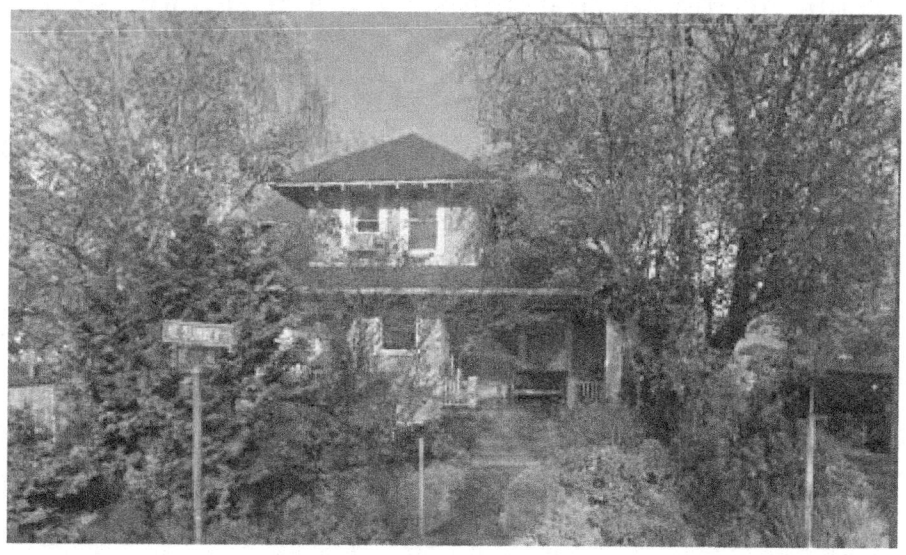

The address of the house was on Sumner Street. The house was right in the middle of where Eleventh Avenue would be if it had gone through. That is where I lived through grade school, high school, and college.

At first, our family lived upstairs, and I had my own bedroom. The house had four prominent dormers.

Each was big enough to be a room, one was a living room, two were bedrooms, one was a kitchen.

That changed as time went on, and our family moved downstairs. Grandma, Auntie Lee, and my father's mother took my upstairs bedroom. I took the downstairs north-east bedroom.

Scooter:
While living in that house, I got a scooter. Now a scooter, for those of you who don't know what a scooter is, is a two-wheeled conveyance-toy, on which you place one foot, push with the other foot, steer with two hands, and brake by stepping on a device that rubs on and stops the front wheel. One can also coast down-hill by putting both feet on the device. Until I wrote this, I never realized how difficult it is to describe in words a thing so simple as a scooter. In any event, my scooter was different. It had eight-inch wheels, rubber tires, and a front brake that would stop the rotation of the front wheel. The problem was that every time I stopped, the front tire would leave a black skid-mart on the riding surface and a flat spot on the tire. I soon had the bumpiest scooter I ever rode, but, boy, could it stop.

Shop:
The basement of Auntie Lee's house was ideal for a shop. It was handy, big, had a concrete floor and a

toilet. My father quit his job at Damascus and put together the room. He painted the basement floor gray to make it easier to clean. He liked the best quality, so a lot of his power tools were made by Delta. He kept adding things until it included: a wood lathe, a swing saw, a jointer, a table saw, a drill press, a metal lathe, a disk sander, a twelve-inch band saw, two used twenty-eight-inch band saws and a five horsepower router.

He built two heavy benches full of drawers and a rack of one hundred and forty-four glass bottles (twelve rows of twelve bottles). The ceiling was made of cardboard stapled to the wooden floor joists and the system and metal hoods for all machines that sawed or made dust. He also made a vacuum. The dirty air was taken out back in a twelve-inch metal pipe, to feed two metal cyclones, mounted in the structure he built. Any air that went out the top of the cyclones went through a water shower to clean them. I never saw such a basement shop. It was awesome. I mention the shop because when my father was done for the day, I often entered the shop to make or fix things.

Streetcars:
I lived during the age of the streetcar. They were not very comfortable, and the conductor did everything while standing. They only had two seats, one on each side of the car. The seats had no springs and ran

lengthwise in the vehicle. The streetcars did have straps for standing passengers, but they ran so often that the straps were seldom used. Most people did not even bother to learn the streetcar's schedule. The worst that could happen was that a potential passenger would have to wait ten minutes for the next streetcar.

Using transfers, which were given out for free upon entering the car, one could ride the streetcars all day for a dime. I never knew anyone who did it, but it was possible.

The cars were made out of wood, so they were relatively cheap. They had steel wheels that traveled on steel tracks that were embedded in the street. Streetcars got their power to travel from a little wheel mounted on a pole that was attached to the top-rear of the car. The power wheel rolled on an overhead wire.

Streetcars could not pull to the curb to take-on or let-off passengers. In fact, the operator could only control the forward speed of the streetcar. The track did all the steering.

I can remember waiting for the streetcar, while standing on the corner of the sidewalk, walking out in the street to the stopped car, getting on the car, and dropping two dimes into the fare collector, then my mental picture fades until we get downtown. I remember getting off the streetcar in the heart of the city and the other passengers heading for their favorite store. Then my memory jumps to an upper floor of a store. We must have waited with a crowd of others for the elevator to arrive.

Elevators are very interesting things. All they do is go up and down, and they are everywhere. What a boring function. That is typical of most machines; they repeat a function over and over until they wear out. Another thing about elevators: No one takes time to read the "Max. Capacity" sign; they just pack it full of people.

My next memory is paying for something. My parents taught me to minimize credit with the saying: When you're out of cash, stop buying! My mother always paid with cash. *(Off topic, but... one time, she took me to the bathroom because I had to go. It was the ladies' room, but I didn't care. Anything was better than wet pants.)*

So much for my typical thought rambling. What was my subject? Oh, yes, streetcars....

Streetcars had two fronts, one at each end. This eliminated any need for an expensive turn-around. All the conductor had to do was remove the speed controller and farebox, walk to the other end of the car and re-install the speed controller handle and farebox, switch power poles and tracks, and he was ready to go. A switch was used to change tracks. The streetcar was not designed to back up, just go forward. Any backing up had to be done by switching ends and going forward the other way.

Photo on a Pony:
When I was about four years old, a man came to the front door selling pictures of a child on a pony. It was not until this writing that I ever wondered why he thought we would ever want such a picture, but he was right--we wanted one. My parents took very few pictures of me. Remember it was in the days of cameras and film. Photos took a lot of time and were expensive. Nowadays, most hand-held electronic devices take digital pictures and are film-less. Even expensive complex cameras take digital photos and are film-less. It turns out that the picture of me on a pony is the only framed picture of me that I have. It didn't take much convincing before my mother said, "Yes." The man dressed me like a cowboy, big hat, chaps, and a toy revolver, and sat me in a saddle on a pony. It was a typically nice day, so the picture was taken on the lawn of the Sumner house, right in front of the living room window and under the Weeping Birch tree.

House Modifications:
After we moved into the Sumner house and were living downstairs, my father took out the heavy wood rolling doors between the living room and the dining room and between the living room and the narthex. The result was that the living room seemed much larger, and the house seemed less dated.

One might think that would have been enough modifications for my parents, but, no, they wallpapered both the living and dining rooms. My father seemed to be the brains behind this whole job. He was still working days for Damascus, but when home, he became The Master Paper-Hanger. He set up a long-narrow aluminum table in the dining room and used it to cut the paper to length and spread the glue. Then he folded the paper, so no glue was on the outside, and carried it to the wall. Starting at the top, he stuck it to the wall. The job went very smoothly, like he was a pro. He, obviously, had done this before.

Chairs and Places:
My parents always had their own living room chairs, and they each had their own living room place. My father's chair was fixed, blue, overstuffed, and located in a corner near the dining area. My mother's chair was a rocker, upholstered with printed flowers, and located near the opening to the dining area. My parents seldom moved furniture. Maybe for

Christmas, but as soon as it was over, things were put back in their places.

I can still mentally picture my father sitting in his chair, eating a raw potato. He liked raw potatoes with a little salt.

Their chairs didn't get used much. They were "doers," not "sitters," as was I, but I also liked to think.

The furnace also had a thermal exit near my mother's chair, which didn't hurt.

The 1940s: A Typical Teenager

I did not go to pre-school or kindergarten but started in the first grade. I went to Highland School (now named Martin Luther King Jr. School) for my elementary schooling. It was a public school and was only about eight blocks away from my house. My mother always fixed me a sack lunch, and I walked. I usually walked alone, went one block south, and then went west on Webster Street because a Doberman on the corner of ninth and Sumner Street scared me. He would follow me along the yard's two-foot-high concrete retaining walk and bark at me. Crossing Sumner Street would take care of the fear of the dog, but then (shh. don't tell anyone) I was afraid of the two old ladies on the other corner. Since I was usually alone and liked it that way, Webster street was the best way to go.

HOW I BECAME ME

There was nothing I feared on that route. There was a worn path across the vacant lot on the corner of 8th and Webster and I usually used it. That got me eighth, on which I went south one block to Alberta, then west on Alberta three blocks, then south about one block to the school. That may sound like a complicated path, but once I figured it out, it was simple, and it only took me a couple days to learn it. I remember when it rained during the day, and I was on my way home from school, water might still be running in the gutter on Eighth Ave. If it were, I'd walk in the gutter and watch a stick or leaf as it floated along. That was fun.

The education people (aka school administration or whatnot) had not yet come up with the concept of a middle school when I attended public school, so I spent eight years at Highland. During my last year there, I was a Crossing Guard. The school provided a three-foot-long dowel, to which a red flag, bearing the word "STOP," was stapled. My job was to hold up the flag whenever kids were in the crosswalk. The hardest part of the job was I had to arrive before the other kids. The best part of the job was stopping the cars. I liked the feeling of power.

My First Bicycle:
I will never forget the day my father picked me up at school and took me to Sears to get me my first

bicycle. I picked a black Elgin with dual headlights, a horn, and a battery. In those days, bicycles only had one speed, and that is what my bike had. It had a double frame, so it was cumbersome. It had balloon tires, which were white walls. The next day my bike was delivered, and I was as proud of it as most kids are today of their first car. It was my ticket to freedom. I must have ridden it over 2,000 miles while I had it. I added a silver wooden box to the back, a brighter headlight powered by a generator, two rearview mirrors, a speedometer, and spray painted it dark green when it got scratched. It lasted through five paper routes, numerous trips to Swan Island, several trips to Rocky Butte, and years of everyday riding. I even learned how to ride it backward, where I would sit on the handlebar and pedal. I never let anyone else ride it, but I think all the kids knew that because no one ever asked. That is kind of ironic because I taught myself to ride a two-wheeler on a borrowed bike. I never used training wheels but would coast by a curb, alone, and not pedal, and I never fell down or in any way damaged the borrowed bike. When I had finished learning, I returned the bike. I think the training bike belonged to a man who had out-grown it. It was like the death of a loved one when I finally sold my bicycle and saw another person ride it off, but that never happened until I got a car.

HOW I BECAME ME

Even today I miss that bike. I bought one from e-bay, assembled it, and tried for over a year to learn to ride it, but I never could. I think I damaged my sense of balance in my fall, so I sold my latest bike, for $2.00, in a garage sale since I couldn't ride it anyway.

War:
The USA was at war with Japan, and I remember the school gym full of bundles of newspapers to aid the war effort. We even had an opaque curtain hanging inside our front door to prevent light from escaping and being used by the Japanese to bomb Portland. Car headlights were taped, so only a slot was uncovered for light to come through. Car speeds were limited to thirty-five miles per hour, even on freeways, to conserve gas. I was never in the military. I was either too young or deferred from being drafted because of schooling. That was good for me because I was adversed at the idea of deliberately hurting another human. I think every human that is born is automatically a citizen of the world. I think it's time to get rid of countries and be one world. It has worked for America, and I think it would work for the world.

Battle Ship Oregon:
This subject is like many others; it is hard to know in which chapter to put it because it happened during my life. I forget when I went on board the battleship Oregon. It was built for WW I, and for a

short time, it was docked in Portland, Oregon, and open to the public as an antique. During that time, I examined the ship. It had been kept in excellent shape far as I could see, with lots of white paint, but at the time, America was into WW II, and to aid in the war effort, the ship was to be scrapped for the metal from which it was made. I later learned that it was not scrapped but became garbage. What an ending for such a ship, and what a waste of white paint.

Food:
During the war, it was hard to get meat. My mother fixed some cuts of meat I have not had since. For example, we had cow tongue, horse meat, and liver. Even though I did not like the taste of tongue, the stringiness of horse meat, nor the look and feel of the uncooked liver, I don't remember anyone ever complaining about what my mother prepared. We always ate meals together in the kitchen around a square table. One of the things that I learned at home and do now is clean my plate. At home, that was drilled into me, and I still do it.

Garage:
I was always kind of a loner. My events relative to the garage is confirmation of that. When the car was gone, and the garage was empty, I used to climb up to the rafters to a hideout. My father had a lot of wood stored up there to air-dry, but there was room

for me. The only problem was the heat during the summer. There was no ventilation, and it was sweaty hot. I never told anybody about it, but it was my secret place. Often during school vacation, I opened the garage's rear window and snitched plums off of the neighbor's tree. I never got caught and really enjoyed eating those plums. (*Please don't rat on me now!*)

Knife thru Window:
One evening I was playing inside, and I decide to throw an unused case knife against the davenport, which was sitting under the front window. The knife went high, bounced off the top of the davenport, and broke the window. The thing I remember most about this event is that neither parent punished me. The window glass was replaced, and no more was ever said about the event. That was the only window I ever broke and the last case knife I ever threw. (*Now, that is real parenting!*)

Dog Pulling Wagon:
We had a Dachshund named Schnapps, and I figured he could pull the wagon with me in it. I tied Schnapps to the wagon, and my younger brother, Bob, ran ahead of the dog, and the dog pulled both me and the wagon. It was an interesting experiment, but I never found any practical use for it. At least I proved that the short-legged dog could pull the wagon with me in it.

FALLING OUT OF NORMAL

Bunk Beds:
My father was great at making things out of wood. He made us a set of bunk beds. Each bed was the same size as a single bed, so if they were ever separated, they could serve as two single beds. He even made a ladder to climb to the top bed and a fence to keep a person safely in the top bed. I took the top bed and used it as long as I lived in the house. He also made two big drawers in each bed. I kept all my comic books in one drawer and my matchbook collection and some clothes in the other. We had matching wall lights for the beds. The problem was finding an outlet. When the house was built, there were not as many electrical items as there were when I lived there. We solved the problem with an extension cord and a plug-strip. We not only had a place to power the lamps, but it supplied power to my radio.

Alarm Clock:
My alarm clock was a wind-up, chime type, Big Ben, and I set it on a chest of drawers my father had made. I can still remember waking up in the top bunk, going to the foot of the bed, rushing down the ladder while pulling the chain which turned on the hanging light in the center of the room, running across the room, and shutting off the alarm clock, then standing still and wondering what time it was. I often took naps on my bed during the day, and I

always set the alarm clock, so I would not be late. There was a moment when I shut off the alarm that I didn't know if my next task was to deliver the morning paper, get ready for school, deliver the afternoon paper, eat dinner, or study. It usually only lasted a moment or so, then I would know what was next. The clock would always whir before it started to chime. The challenge was to shut it off before it chimed. I never made it, but I came close. Hardly anything was battery-powered in those days. Most had to be wound. I was too young to have a watch, but most of them had to be wound every day. They ran all day on one winding, but not two days.

Buried Box:
One day I became the possessor of a big wooden box. By big, the inside dimensions were like 7x7x7 feet. I decided it would make a great playhouse, and buried it would be even better. My parents didn't object, so in the lot next to our house, I dug a hole big enough to hold the box. I put the box in the hole and covered all but an access port with dirt. The only trouble with the buried house was that I never got around to playing in it. Eventually, it got filled with tree and grass clippings. At least nobody fell into the box. That could really hurt.

A Model:
My father had quit his job at Damascus Milk Company and was making the wooden part of

wooden shoes in the basement shop. I was the only boy at Highland who wore wooden shoes to school. I liked them because they kept my feet dry and because they could be re-soled and re-heeled without having to give up a new shoe coupon, which was demanded by the Federal Government as a war aid. They were very popular with men who worked on a wet floor, like a dairy.

The only problem I ever found with them was carelessly stepping on a rock. If one was not alert, they could turn an ankle. It never happened to me, but it could happen.

The wood part of the wooden shoe was band-sawed out of a block of Alder.

My father had bought the empty lot next to the house, which he used to air dry Alder planks. The planks were then cut into blocks and band sawed into shoe bottoms. The band sawing produced an unwanted Alder "skeleton," which was thrown into a large box built by my father out of half-inch plywood and mounted on casters for easy moving. I sold the boxes full of dry Alder skeletons to the neighbors delivered for twenty cents as fire-starters.

That accomplish four things:
1. It emptied the boxes
2. It gave the neighbors an excellent fire starter

3. It got me out of his hair for a while
4. It gave me a little money

I remember the day I was called out of class by the gym teacher who was trying to convince a boy to wear wooden shoes home because that is all she had that would fit him. It must have worked because the boy put on the shoes and I went back to class.

Home Made Kites:
I must have made twenty of my own diamond-shaped kites. I bought the string and used it to tie the horizontal stick to the vertical rod, bow the horizontal stick, make the bridle, tie it to the vertical stick, and then tether the line. I covered them with newspaper and with a stabilizing tail. They flew great!

My biggest homemade kite was six feet tall, but it was not my best flyer. It kept trying to lift me off the ground.

They were not very colorful, being covered with old newspaper, but they were cheap.

Target Kite:
I even bought a war surplus blue nylon covered kite. It was originally designed to be a target kite and had a picture of a Japanese Zero painted on it. That kite had no tail and was intended to be unstable. It was

flown on two lines attached on the ground to two drums about two feet apart and mounted on a stick or rod. On the kite end, the lines were fastened to a rudder mounted on the bottom of the vertical. By pulling on one line while relaxing the other, the kite could be made to dart right or left. The task of the shooter was to hit the darting kite. Obviously, these kites were expendable.

Yo-Yo's:
I was awesome with a Duncan yo-yo: I had two of them, a red one and a blue one. They were both made of wood, as were all yo-yo's in those days. Mine was carved by me and made very personal. I practiced until I could do most of the yo-yo tricks. The most dangerous trick was "Around The World." The first time I did it, the string broke, and the yo-yo went flying. I quickly learned to only do that trick on a new or almost new string.

Recently I bought a couple of yo-yos designed to make some tricks easier, but I have lost whatever skill I had, confirming the saying: USE IT OR LOSE IT.

Just look at what I use for skill now. None.

Grandfather's Snare Drum:
One day I found my grandfather's snare drum. Finding his drum and Auntie Lee's remarks really

inspired me to become a drummer, so I took lessons. My teacher came to the house and brought with him a practice pad mounted on a drum stand. He directed me to practice on the pad so as not to make others be blasted by the sound of a drum. I practiced on the pad for about a year, then I got a real snare drum. I joined the Highland orchestra as a snare drummer and never regretted it.

Tree Climbing:
Few rules went with living in the house, but the rule I violated the most was, "Don't climb the weeping birch tree in the front yard." That tree was just screaming to be climbed. Auntie Lee never offered a reason for the rule, so I just waited until no one was around, and I climbed clear to the top. I never got caught nor discovered the reason for the rule.

Games:
I played a lot of softball after school. We usually played in the street at the intersection of 11th. And Webster. We never had enough kids to have teams, so we used rotation. The sidewalk corners were our bases, with the south-west corner being home. Most of my games were outside ones, softball, basketball, kick-the-can, hide-and-seek, like those.

Furnace Change:
When we moved in, the house was heated by gravity and burned sawdust. For years sawdust was

dumped and stored adjacent to the basement window. I used to shovel the sawdust through the window into the storage room. The sawdust was then shoveled into a huge metal hopper and gravity-fed it into the burner. Every couple of hours, someone had to go downstairs and fill the hopper, or the fire would go out. The old furnace was replaced by an oil furnace, and life got easier. The heated air was then move by a fan, which meant the ducts could be much smaller than the gravity ducts.

The oil storage tank was buried in the front yard as part of the furnace installation.

Bird:
For a while, we had a small multi-colored bird kept in a cage in the dining room. Not being a canary, it never sang. I never liked the bird very much, but since it existed, I had to tolerate it. I never found out who bought it, but I suspected it was my mother. I even tried talking to the bird, but to no avail; it just sat on a perch and stared at me.

Dogs:
It seems that as long as we live downstairs in the Sumner house, we had dogs, but they were always of the small breed type. The first one I remember was the Boston Bulldog. He was very little trouble, but not much fun either. Mostly he kept to himself. I don't even remember his name. We had him for a

long time, but he turned yellow and died. I now suspect it was some kind of liver disease.

He was followed by a Dachshund named Schnapps. He was a lot more fun than the Bulldog, but it might have been my age. I was older by the time Schnapps joined the family. I made him a signal to have a human open the back door and let him in. The backyard was fenced, and he was often let out into the backyard to piddle or poop. The signal to let him in was an electric buzzer inside switched on. When the dog pawed at the spring-loaded board, the back door opened. Pushing the board with his paws closed a switch, which rang the buzzer. He was quick to learn how it worked and used it for years.

Another trick of his was to hoof it two blocks to the butcher shop on Alberta Street and get a big bone. The bone was often too large for Schnapps to get up the curb to the sidewalk, forcing him to walk in the street on his return trip to the house. He was not about to put the bone down. It might be snatched by another dog.

Bottles on a Rack:
One of the things I learned from my father was how to make a rack of bottles for sorting and storing things. First, get a lot of small glass containers. I got 144, wide mouth, three inches tall, glass bottles. They can be divided into twelve rows of twelve

bottles each. Second, build a solid backed rack of twelve shelves, a half-inch wider than the diameter of a bottle, a half-inch further apart than the height of a bottle, and a quarter-inch longer than the diameters of twelve bottles. Add ends and a top equal to the width of the bottom shelf. Add a strip to the front of each shelf so the bottles won't fall off the shelves. This shelf unit can be hung on a wall and will give you 144 places to store things that take little space, are visible, and are easy to retrieve. I know. I made one.

Newspaper Routes:

At one time, I had two paper routes. (Shh. -That is I had a delivery route for each of the two competing newspapers in Portland, Oregon. I knew this was a no-no for each of the newspaper companies, so I didn't tell anyone--except for you now.) One paper was delivered early in the morning, and the other in the evening, so there was no conflict for me. The papers were rolled into a cylinder shape, tucked into themselves, put in a bag, which was mounted on the handlebars of a bicycle. The papers were delivered by throwing them on the porch so they wouldn't get wet. Each company had the same rules for a delivery person. The job could be divided into three parts: deliver the paper, collect the payments from the delivery of that month, and paying the monthly bill. It was often hard to get people to pay. The rest was easy.

HOW I BECAME ME

Shack Manager:
I stayed with the morning newspaper, The Oregonian, long enough to become a shack manager. The job of a shack manager was to open the paper shack, build a fire in the stove if it was cold outside, break open the paper bundles that were delivered, and give each carrier the number of papers he needed to cover his route. The routes varied in size, from twenty to sixty customers, so I had to learn the number of papers to give each carrier. Not only that, but the number of customers on any route might vary on a day-to-day basis, so it was a never-ending job situation.

The shack was heated by a small sheet-metal stove that burned papers. I would stuff the rolls of paper into the stove and light it. Often the stove would get red hot, but it never caught the shack on fire. I had to get up at 3:30 a.m. to keep that job. I had a fifty-customer route, one of the bigger routes, which I delivered to each weekday morning. The newspaper truck usually arrived by 4:00 a.m. and delivered bundles of 100 papers tied by wire. It was my job to cut the wire and distribute. The carriers would roll, then tuck the papers into themselves, and put them in a bag. The bag was then put on the handlebar of the bike and secured, thereby "S" shaped hooks that went inside the handlebar ends and held the bag on the bike. The carrier was then ready to ride around his route, throwing the papers on the dry porches.

Screen Door:
One morning, as I was delivering the papers, I hit one of my customers front screen doors. The hit was hard enough to completely destroy the screen. Later in the day, I agreed to fix the screen, but the customer balked at the idea of me fixing it. He believed only a professional could get the screen tight. I agreed to let him be the judge, either my fix or I would pay to have a pro. Try to fix it, he relented. Later that same day, I returned with my fix, and my customer was greatly impressed with how tight the screen was. Then I told him that my father had been making screens for some time, and he got the screen tight by stapling the screen to the bottom board, bending the sideboards with clamps, pulling the screen as tight as possible by hands, and stapling the screen to the top board, then removing the clamps and stapling the screen to the sideboards. The customer said that the door was like new. We both left happy.

Elementary Student:
I was never a very good student. C was my usual grade. On the other hand, I never failed, so at least I graduated. I got tired of being asked what I wanted to be when I grew up. Finally, in desperation, I said,

"a physicist." I am not sure they knew what that meant, but it stopped the questioning.

Caves:

I was no spelunker, but I liked Rocky Butte and its caves. I often rode there on my bicycle. The caves were about halfway up, and they were great to explore. I was too chicken to go very far, but I went far enough to be entertained. The view from the top of the butte was spectacular, and the coast down on my bike was fun.

The 1950s: I was a Big Drip. You Dig?

Jefferson High School:
I graduated from Highland and went to Jefferson High School. I joined the Jef band. It got me into all the high school games free and into all the parades. It even got me a ride on a police motorcycle. The Jefferson High School band was scheduled to perform during halftime for a Rose Bowl football game, but no one had thought to bring the drumsticks. I volunteered to go with the policeman back to the school to get the drumsticks. We went by motorcycle. My only ride on such a beast, but we made it in time, and none of the spectators knew what had happened.

Photo Lab:
I made my own photo lab. There was a closet off the main floor hall under the stairs to upstairs that was big enough for a small photo lab. All I had to do was add a red light and a wide shelf. For a while, photography was a big thing for me. I made enlargements of any negative I could get.

Snow Skiing:
Laurence (Andy) Anderson and Auntie Lee were married by then and lived upstairs. Andy built a cabin at Government Camp on Mount Hood, and it was there that I learned to snow ski. My first pair of skis were wood, long, and army surplus. I even trail-skied with them from Timberline Lodge to Government Camp several times. I later got a pair of used fiberglass skis, which were shorter, lighter, and had quick-release binders. The new skis were much easier to handle. I never got very good at snow skiing, but I enjoyed it.

The Bowling Alley:
For a while, I worked in a bowling alley setting pins. That was before the machine pinsetter was invented. It was the dirtiest job I ever had. Every time the ball hit the back-pit pad, it gave off a cloud of dirt. Some of that dirt would get on the pinsetter. I usually went home with a smudged-stained face. The money was not very good either—only ten cents a line (a line was ten frames long). Occasionally I set

two lanes at once, but it increased the probability of being hit by a flying pin, or worse yet, a ball. If things were very slow, the pinsetters would bowl, but they always played "low man sets." Since I usually had to set, I gave up bowling with them.

Some bowlers throw a very fastball with a lot of spin on it. This tends to shorten the time it takes to bowl a line but increases the probability of being hit by a flying pin, and the ball hits the back-pit pad harder, causing more dirt.

Tall Christmas Tree:
I will never forget the big Christmas tree my father bought. He always bought the tree, and most of them fit fine, but one year he went crazy. He purchased a tree that must have been sixteen feet tall. Our home ceiling must have been eight feet or less. We cut one foot off the bottom and about seven feet off the top. It was the biggest and fullest home tree I ever saw. The base of the tree trunk was four inches in diameter. Wow, what a tree.

Asbestos Siding:
Sometime during this period, Auntie Lee decided to have asbestos siding put on the house. The asbestos shingles were very brittle, and although held in place by nails, the shingles were too abrasive to drill holes, so the application team used a special hole punch to make holes in the shingles for the nails. The nails

needed to be driven in until they held the shingle in place, but any extra hammering could shatter the shingle. They were very talented at driving nails. Over sixty years later, when I saw the house, it still looked good. There was no sign of decay, and though it had not been done, the asbestos could be painted if an owner wanted to change the color of the house.

U Control Models:

I became very interested in model airplanes as a teenager, particularly building and flying U control models. For those who are not aware of U control, it is an airplane model with a wingspan of two feet or less, usually powered by a small gas engine, and flown in a circle around the pilot on two thin sixty-feet long wires that control the pitch of the elevator. I joined a club and eventually became president of it. Like everything, technology advanced and produced the glow plug, so the engine ran like a diesel engine, the pressure regulator, so the engine would run at any altitude, and the plastic U Rely so the pilot could easily change the length of the wires. Clyde, my best friend, and an avid U control pilot, later became my brother-in-law. We flew our airplanes at night in the rain and in the snow with a flashlight fastened to the bodies of the structures. We even flew in the wind, making lazy-eights on the downwind side of the circle to keep the control wires tight. I built a model that handled as well upside as it did right side up. It was great for lazy-eights.

My First Car:
I bought my first car from Wade Helzer, who was going into the Navy. He had to sell his black 1933 Ford sedan. It had a V8 engine and a 4.11 rear end, so its acceleration was great, but it also had mechanical brakes, so its ability to stop was questionable. I use to hunt the auto wrecking yards. It was in one of those yards that I found a full set of 1940 Ford hydraulic brakes that could eliminate the '33 Ford stopping problem. I bought them, installed them, and had no more problems. I spent a lot of money on that car, what with new upholstery, moon hubcaps, new dash cover, and new shocks, but it was worth it.

Roofing:
It was after I got the car that I became a roofer. Paul Natero was my boss/teacher. He installed new asphalt roofing over whatever material was used before. He was swamped with orders and needed help. I used the apprentice concept; I watched and learned. Paul was a great teacher, and I was a fast learner. We attached the new material with galvanized nails, driving them with a hatchet. Paul paid me $2.75 for every square I put on and $3.00 for pitched roofs. The hardest part of the roofing job was carrying the new material from the ground,

where it was unloaded, up the ladder to the old roof. It was a great job, though. And I made enough to support my car and start college.

Meeting My Wife:
One day, as I was walking up the front steps of Clyde's house, I noticed a girl on a blanket in the front yard. I asked him, "Who is that?" He said, "Oh, she is my sister. She has been away at school." I learned later that her name was Joyce, and she was attending North West Nazarene College in Idaho. She later declared, "I will never marry a man who is *not* a Christian." So I became a Christian.

I joined the Nazarene church and did some stupid things. For example, Joyce had a fit when she saw me arrive to a service wearing the wrong pants. This resulted in almost getting kicked out of the church!! I had been snow-skiing all day, and I showed up to church with my ski pants on. (I had never been raised in any church. In fact, I had never seen my father inside any church. My mother was not a member of any church. My parents taught me about honesty and truth but didn't use a church to teach lessons on ethics and morals.)

Dating:
Before long, I was dating Joyce. A typical date was driving her to Janzen Beach, parking near the fence,

climbing on top of the car, and looking over the fence to watch the midget autos race. Talk about a cheap date! That must hold some kind of a record. My only cost was gas to drive there and back, and gasoline was cheap then. I didn't date many girls (maybe two). Doris was my other girlfriend, but she kept interfering with my U control flying, so I dropped her.

Gas Station:
I worked in the Texaco gas station on the south-east corner of 11th and Alberta Street. I liked cars, and there I saw lots of them. Oregon is one of the few states where the driver can't legally pump gas—station-man can do that. I have no proof, but I think it was a safety measure. A station-man presumably knows gasoline is inflammable and never smokes around a fire. I see pumping gas while smoking often in Washington state.

Another thing I want to point out about the old days: when a driver stopped for gas, the windshield and headlights got cleaned, and the ashtray got emptied. Some stations even vacuumed the front floor. That kind of service no longer exists, but it did in my time.

Desk:
I needed a study desk in my bedroom, so I made one. It was just a piece of plywood on two cabinets, but

it served my needs. Little did I know until I went to Boeing that they had done the same things, only the top was bigger, and the cabinets were taller. I used that desk for high school and college studies.

22 Caliber Pistol:
My father liked to shoot and bought himself a 22 caliber automatic pistol. He always kept it loaded and hanging in a holster on his bed headboard. I knew it was there but never touched it. He always took it camping. On one camping trip, he even let me shoot it. That was the only time I ever shot it. I don't know what became of that pistol.

32 Caliber Revolver:
When my father returned from WW I, he brought a 32 caliber silver revolver and a box of shells. As a curious teenager, I tore the gun apart to see how it worked. During the reassembly, I discovered that I had lost the key to align the cylinder with the barrel so the bullet will enter it and the gun will not explode in your hand. I always intended to have a gunsmith make a new key and put it in the gun, but I never did, so I never fired it. I later learned after my son took the gun to a gunsmith that not only was the key missing, but the barrel had been expanded, probably by one bullet stopping in the barrel and the second bullet being fired and running into the first one. His recommendation "Don't ever fire the gun."

OH, BTW:
A drip is a slang word we used in the 1950s for someone who was very uncool. *You dig* means: do you understand? You can also say, *you catch my drift?*

The 1960s & 70s: Building a Life (and a House)

My Future:
In 1951, I was still in college, but my future looked very bleak; I didn't have enough money for my last year. Student loans had not been invented yet, and I was unable to come up with any funding source. Then, out of the blue and without any contract, Auntie Lee loaned me $200. I was able to stay in college and graduate. Years later, I gave her the borrowed $200. She was surprised. She always thought she was giving me a gift. I guess the loan idea was mine. I think $200 sounds like a trivial amount because today it would be, but with inflation, it would be like $2,000 now—anyway, her "gift" of $200 allowed me to stay in school and graduate.

HOW I BECAME ME

1952:
1952 was a big year for me. While I was still in college, with Physics as my major, I was hired by a Boeing representative named Roughner. I moved out of the childhood house, which I always thought of as my home, to Seattle. I got married to Joyce in a Nazarene Church. I graduated from Portland University with a BS in Physics. We honeymooned on the Olympic Peninsula in a cabin on a lake. My father had loaned me his 1941 Oldsmobile, one of the first autos to have an automatic transmission, so I had no car trouble.

Boeing:
For thirty-two years, I spent most of my adult life working for Boeing in Military Products. I went on over 200 trips for them, and they made all the reservations for me and paid for everything. They turned me from a Physicist into an Engineer, and it only took them about a week. I remember one time being asked: "Are you a Mechanical or an Electrical Engineer?" My answer was: "Yes." My first job with Boeing required calculus, but most of the work I did for Boeing was as a Systems Engineer whose job was to be sure things worked together. To that end, I made a lot of Interface Control Drawings. I never was a manager but was classed as an individual contributor, and that was fine with me.

BOMARC:

I worked on Boeing Michigan Aerospace Research Center (BOMARC) for years while the Hamilton Watch Company (HWC), located in Lancaster, PA, designed, built, and tested the only purple unit in the missile, the warhead Safety and Arming Programmer. The BOMARC missile was designed to be launched from the ground storage building, which had a split roof. With the roof open, the missile could be erected vertically outside the building and launched. They had a test launcher near the Boeing 2.01 building. It was a sunny Saturday morning when I was walking past the Boeing test launcher building on my way to work. I heard a rumble and thought that's funny, it didn't even look like rain. Then I saw it, the launcher roof was opening. As the missile came out of the building, I realized I WAS TOO CLOSE. I'D BE BURNED ALIVE BY THE ROCKET ENGINE. It only lasted a few seconds, and I almost wet my pants!! Thank goodness, it was just a test, and there was no rocket motor ignition. Boy, was I frightened! (BTW: It was from the Watch Division of the HWC that I bought a wristwatch for my wife.)

Amish:

During my visits to the HWC, I was able to see real Amish people. Mostly they kept to themselves, but often I encountered a horse-drawn buggy on the road. They didn't even have a church building but met weekly in members' homes. The married women, married men, unmarried boys, and unmarried girls were segregated. I never saw a woman and man together except for if they were married to each other.

ALCM:
After BOMAC, I worked on the Air-Launched Cruise Missile (ALCM). It was designed to be carried on the B-52. Eight missiles were carried in the bomb bay on a rotary launcher, and six missiles were mounted on pylons under each wing, for a total of twenty missiles per B-52. The wings, elevators, and engine air intake were folded to reduce the carriage size of the missile and unfolded after launch. The Williams company built the engine for the ALCM. The ALCM is still operational at this writing even though the B-52 is over fifty years old. I made many trips to make sure that the engine met all of its requirements.

IUS:
After ALCM, I worked on the Interim Upper Stage (IUS), which was a thrust stage that could be added to a Minute Man missile to increase its range. It was on that program that I got to go inside of one of the operational missile launch sites. The whole site was mounted on large coiled springs so it wouldn't be knocked out by an enemy's near-miss or an earthquake. Security was very high on the site. I was

one of the few non-military people that ever got to enter an operational Minute Man missile site.

Motor Vehicles:
I liked cars and at one time had fourteen motor vehicles. They included a GMC RV, a '48 Dodge pickup, a small motorcycle, an XK 120 1952 Jaguar Roadster, and several Cadillac limousines. Nowadays, cars are controlled by computers, and I can't even fix them. It takes special test equipment to determine what is wrong. I don't have that equipment. In the old days, I used to rebuild engines when they needed it. That is part of my past. I just passed my eighty-eighth birthday, and I am still going strong. Most people die before then.

Water Ski:
I learned to water ski. I got so good at it I could single-ski. My father had moved out of the basement and into a much larger place. He made wooden skies for Lauderback, who put on the binders and sold the finished ski. Father also made me a fourteen-foot-long plywood boat. I bought a twenty-five horsepower outboard engine and a lot on Lake Cavanaugh, and I was set to go. I never tried jumping, but I had fun skiing. I even taught a young boy how to make a deep water start on a single ski. The boy suffered the loss of control of his left leg from polio. I got him on top of the water by straddling his single ski between my two skies, and

when he got up, I let go. It only took a couple of spills before he could stay up, but he finally made it.

My House:

One day I got the bright (and crazy) idea that I should build a house. I could incorporate all my great ideas into its design, and it would be fun. Little did I know what building a house would involve. I had never built one before but assumed I could do it. I am not talking about being a contractor; I am talking about building a house with my own two hands, like driving nails and laying bricks. I found a floor plan I liked in a magazine. The design was by Frank Lloyd Wright. How could I go wrong with Frank? I would need to reverse the floor plan to fit the lot and incorporate my ideas. The upstairs would be about two thousand square feet and downstairs the same, for a total of four thousand square feet. Then I bought a book titled Architects Graphic Standard, which gave things like the rise and run of stairs, location of light switches, and other code data and I was all set.

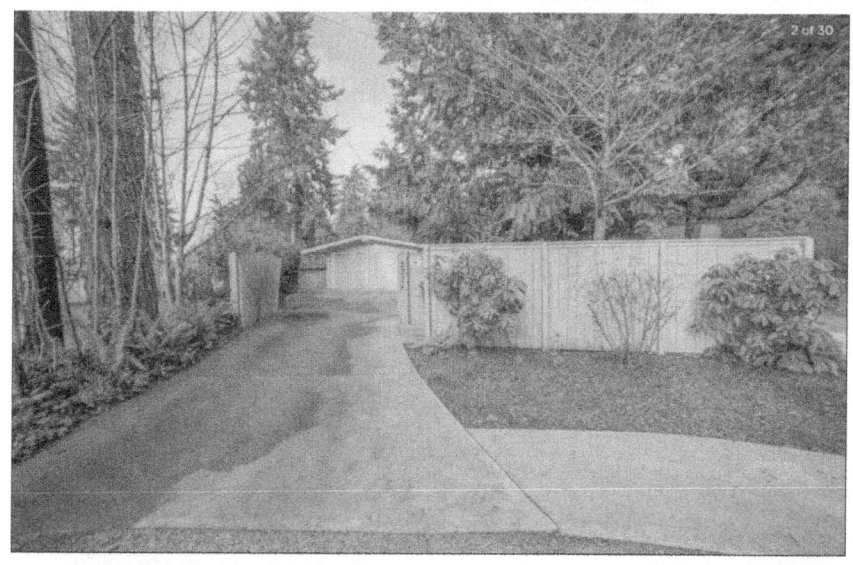

Lot:
I bought an acre lot in Federal Way, WA, that fit my ideas. It was high, no water problems, on a cul-de-sac, no traffic noise, east of the commercial airplane flight path, no airplane engine noise, wooded, fuel for heat if the furnace fails, covered with the natural ground cover, no yard maintenance, it even had a small creek.

Roof Design:
The house was designed to have an open ceiling. The main beam running the length of the building was a rough sawed eight by eighteen. The rafters were rough sawed twelve inches tapering to six inches by fours on eight-foot centers. The connections between the central bean and each rafter were made by a two-foot-long steel tube. Each steel tube passes through the center of the central beam and into the

ends of opposite rafters. The ceiling was made of eight-foot-long two by six tongue and grooved then beveled planks stained white. That made a solid roof. The central beam was notched 1/4 inch deep on each side where the rafters met the primary beam to allow it to shrink as it dried.

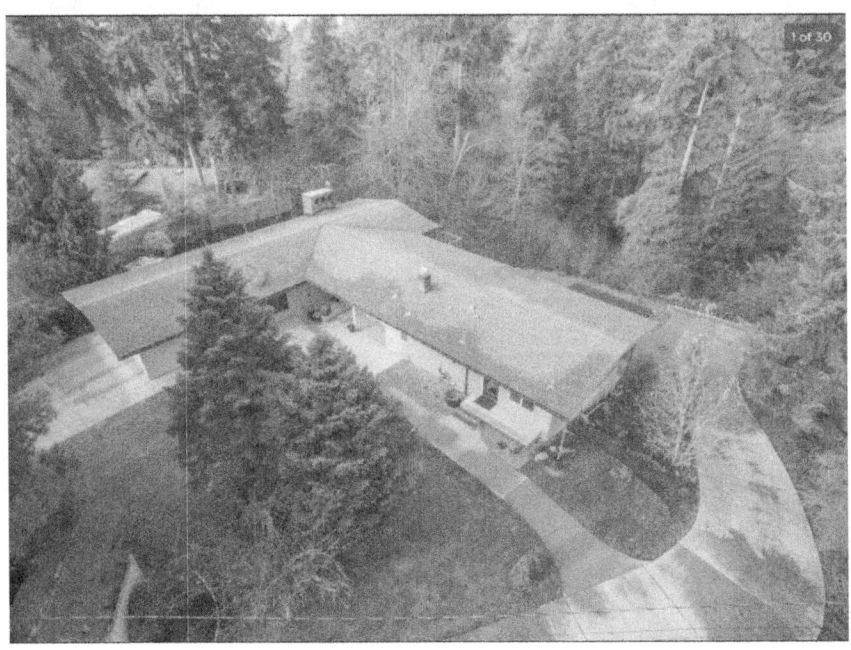

It was while I was in high school that I became a roofer. I learned how to asphalt a roof by watching Paul Natero do it. He was a pro at it.

In those days, one man did everything. Nowadays it takes five or six men to do what one man did, not only that but the new material is now set on the roofing by machine whereas in my days as a roofer the new roofing material was carried one half a bail at a time from the ground up the ladder to the roof, by hand. The hatchet and nails have been replaced by staples that are driven by compressed air. So I do not qualify as a roofer anymore. That is fine with me. I don't plan to reroof anything at the present time.

Drawings:

My next task was to make drawings. My job at Boeing was to make Interface Control Drawings, so house drawings were right up my alley. I produced about six 24 x 48 drawing sheets, fastened them to a stick, rolled them up, and headed for the building permit office. They liked my drawings, but it had omitted plumbing, so it was back to the drawing board to make a plumbing drawing. On my second trip, I got a building permit, and I was ready to go.

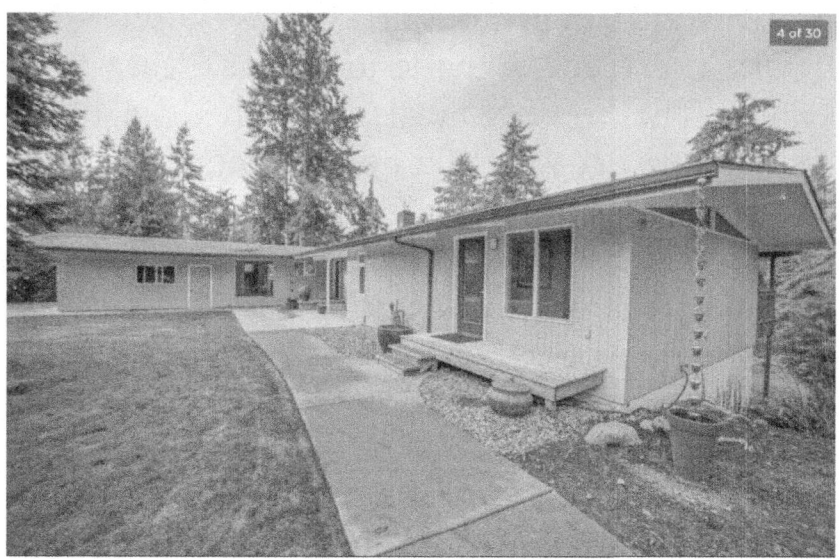

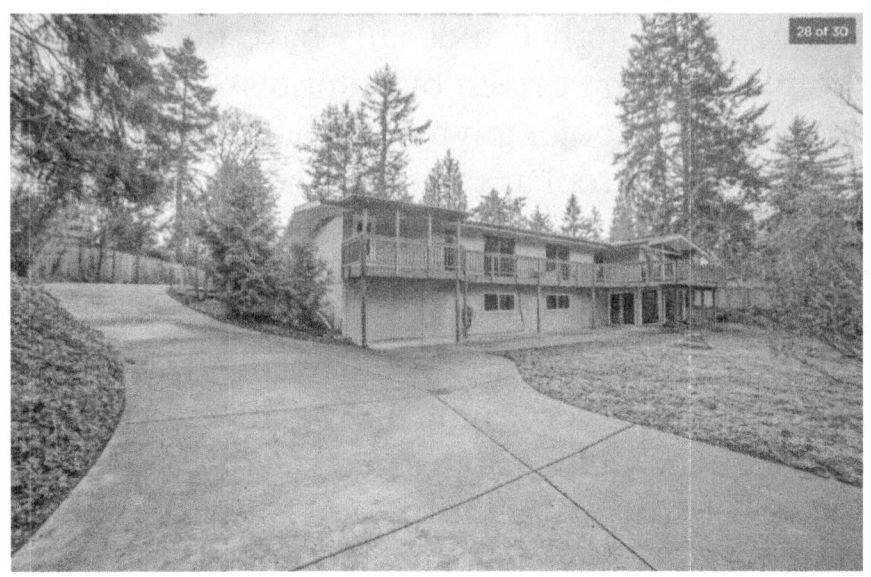

Design:

The house was designed to support two families: one downstairs and one upstairs. It even had separate front doors and driveways. Later when I had built the fence, I made a separate gate for the basement. The house was also designed for fire and earthquake. Every room had exits on opposite sides, so one could get out in case of fire. The house was also designed to stay in one piece in case of an earthquake. The ground could shake, but the house would not fracture.

Concrete:

Putting up the forms for the concrete walls of the basement was a big job. The forms were made of half-inch plywood held apart by metal rods and washers. The upper floor would be about three feet above the ground, and the lower floor or basement would be about five feet below the ground. I had shoveled the dirt out of the lower part so the basement could be formed. The concrete truck arrived and flowed concrete into the forms, and the basement walls were made. After the concrete had been set up, the forms were removed, and the outside of the walls was painted with tar to prevent any wall water from getting into the basement. The basement floor was also concrete, but it was laid on a bed of gravel covered by a sheet of plastic to drain any groundwater.

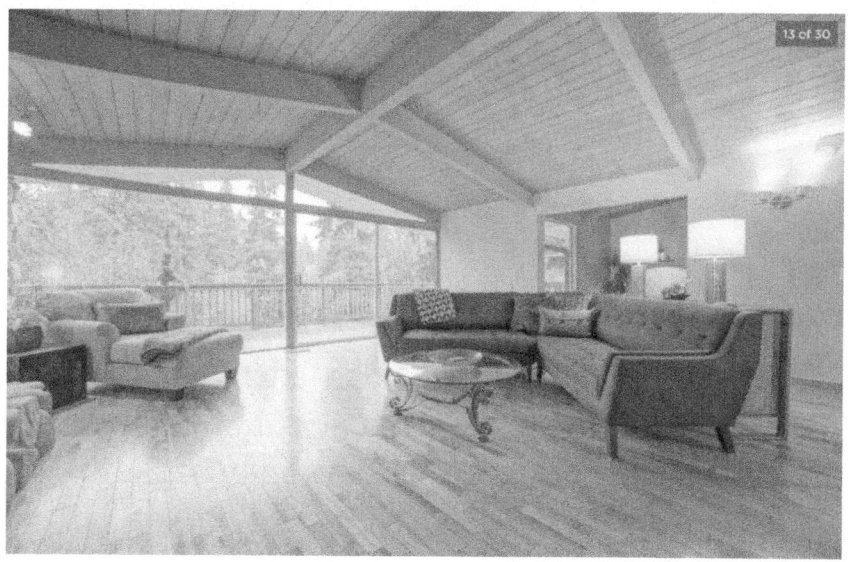

Help:
I did hire some help on framing, window glass, the furnace, roofing, concrete troweling, and waste plumbing. The waste plumbing help, however, was free and was provided by my cousin Tommy who was training to be a licensed plumber.

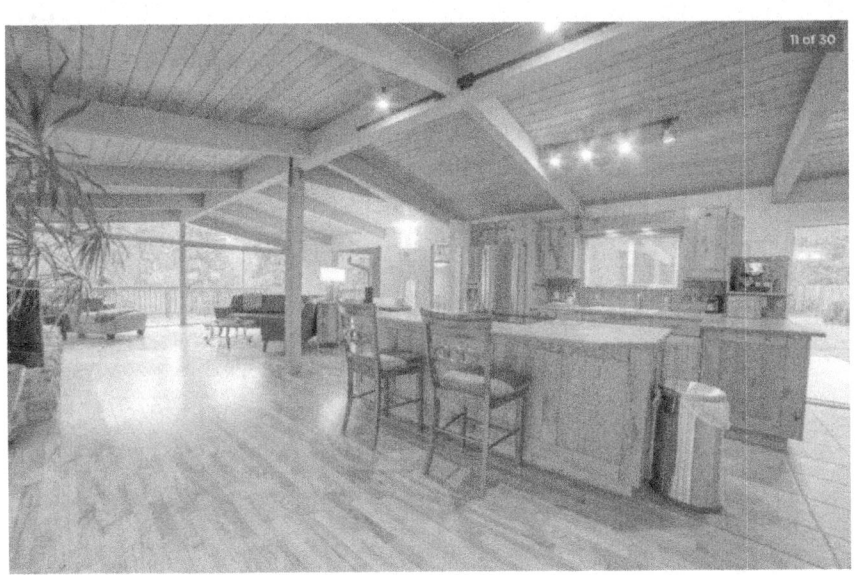

Roof, Siding & Floor:
On the weather side, I used solid sheets of insulation over the planks, then tar paper, then hot mop, then gravel. The siding was vertical tongue and groove cedar boards stained dark brown. The upstairs floor was mostly made up of old form plywood with the concrete side turned down. The exception to that was near the kitchen, where I intended to one day add stone but never got around to it.

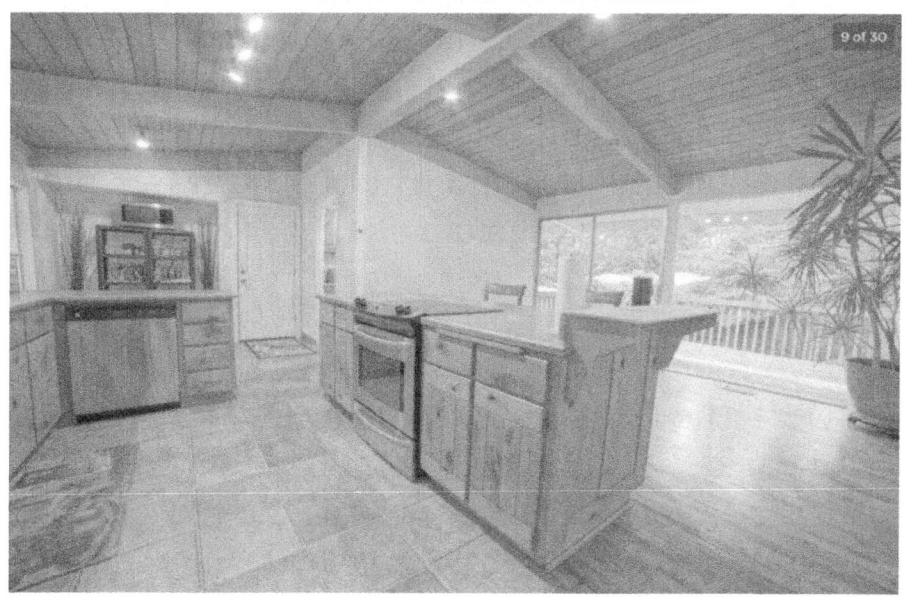

Brick Laying:
The house was finally livable, at least the downstairs was, so we moved in. I had walled off the west end of the basement, and that is where we lived. The furnace had not been installed yet, so we heated with the fireplace. It was the largest fireplace I had ever seen. It could take a six-foot-long log and had dual flues and chimneys. The sidewalls of the fireplace were built at an angle to better heat the room. I learned how to lay bricks from building the upstairs and downstairs fireplaces. All the fireplace chimneys were capped by a cement cap to prevent down drafting.

Septic System:
The septic tank was the largest built at the time, a thousand gallons, big enough to handle two families.

I dug the hole, and the tank was lowered into it by crane. The system had a distribution box and three laterals. It was on a hillside where no machine could work, so I dug it all by hand. I put in the gravel, pipe, tar paper, and back covered it all.

A New Roof:

Only two rooms in the house ever got finished, and they were the upstairs bathroom and kitchen. By then, we had moved upstairs and had four kids, but we still had cardboard doors on all the kid's rooms. Why did the house never get finished? My wife was a hoarder, and things got so full of stuff I could no longer get to the places that needed work and rather than insisting that stuff be moved, I gave up, but not until I reroofed the house with three-tab black asphalt shingles because the old roof started to leak.

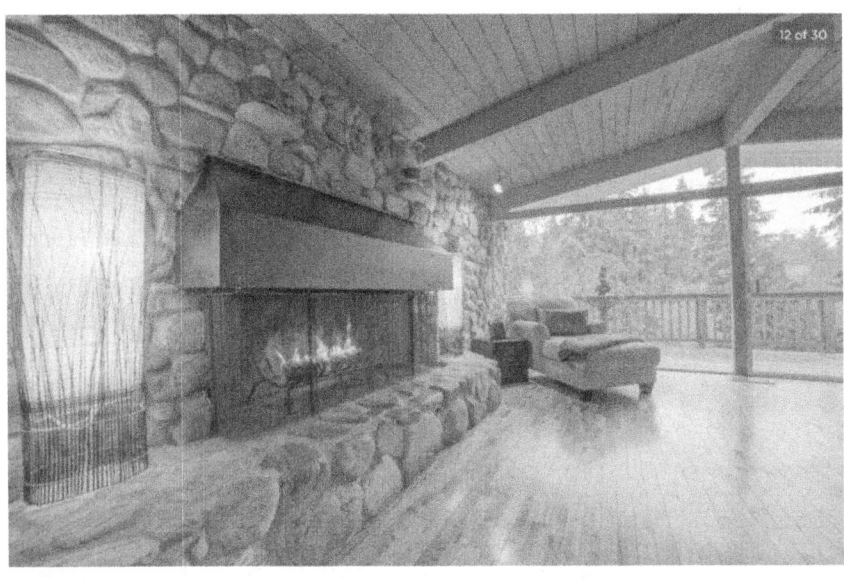

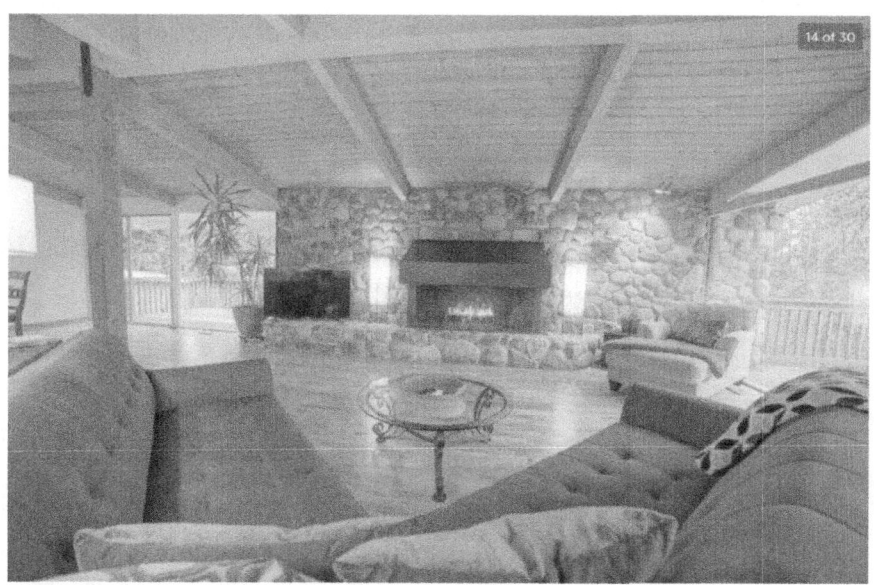

Alarm System:

I am no longer interested in hang gliding. I just passed my eighth-eighth birthday and still going strong. I live with my daughter, and she is still keeping me supplied with all my needs. I no longer have a house of my own. I often wonder what the present house-owner did with the indoors alarm system. The whole system was inside the house.

Lower Level:

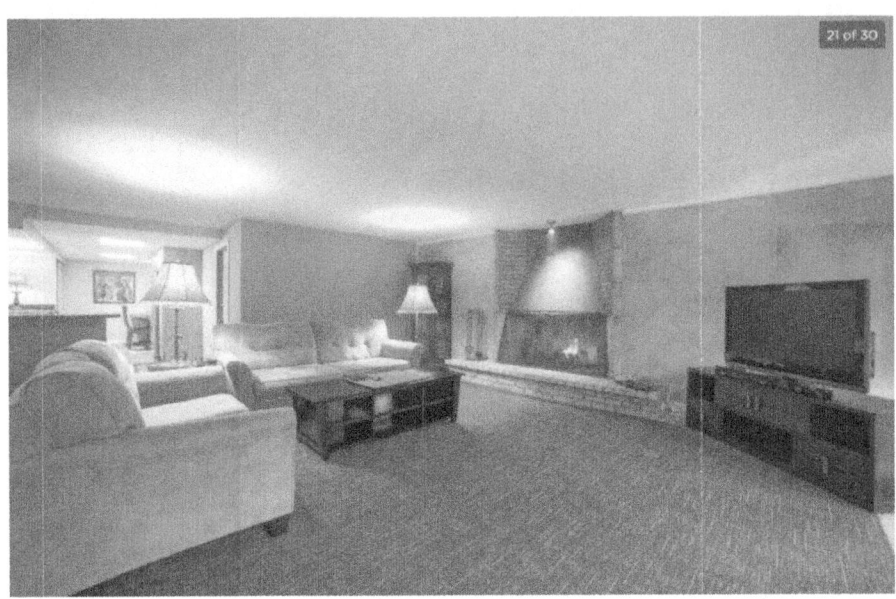

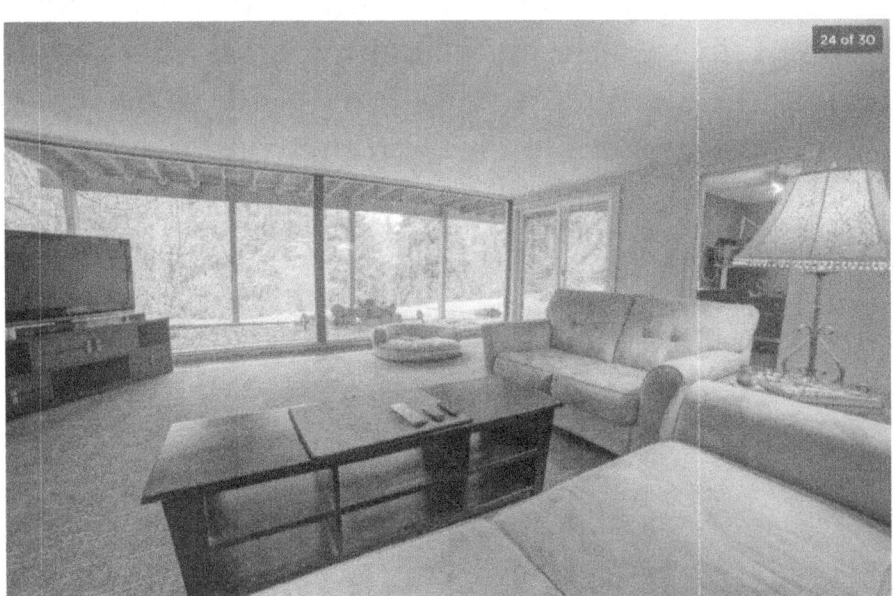

Second Kitchen:

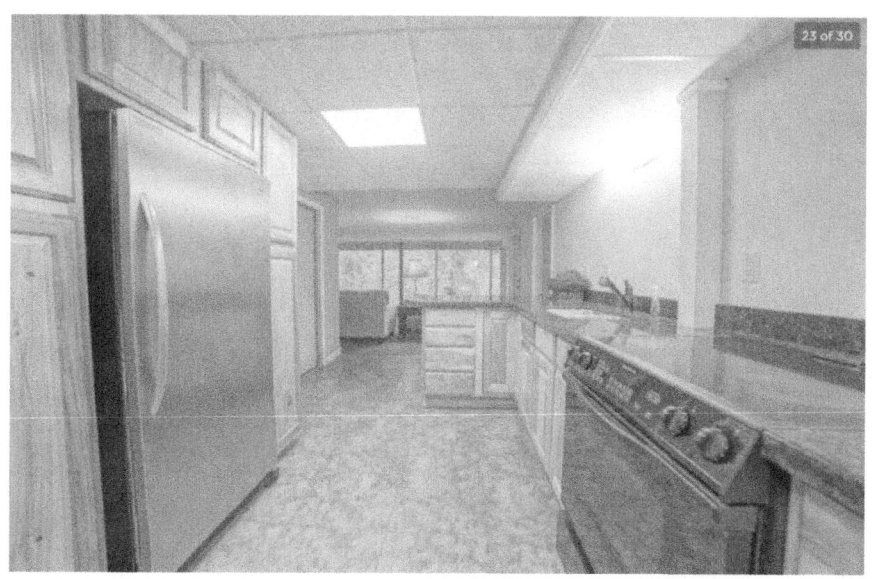

My Home:

I never got to live in the house I designed and started building even after it was finished because of my injury. The photos are from a real estate site. I just got to see the pictures after a stranger finished my project. This is the hardest part about being "disabled." I was removed from my home after my injury, and then unable to afford to purchase it back after it had been placed on the real estate market. Sometimes, when you're "disabled" (and even when you're not), you are forced to let go of your wishes and dreams.

The 1980s: Falling Out of Normal

"I don't suffer from insanity. I enjoy every moment of it."
- Allen

It all got started by Lyon McCandless, a fellow Boeing employee. He had been doing it for years without incident and told me how easy it was to learn. –

He liked the thrill of flying like a bird over the ground and trees. As a person gets more proficient as a pilot, he can fly into a thermal, which is raising air caused by ground heat and stay aloft for a long time. Asphalt or a plowed field could always cause thermals by late in the afternoon if the sun heated them. Old-timers would not fly until late in the day because that was when the thermals got formed.

They would also watch the large birds. They could smell the warmed air and inform the experienced pilots where the thermals were.

As a novice, I did not look for thermals. My flights were all "sled rides" or still air flights.

My wife, Joyce, didn't like me hang gliding. She thought it was too dangerous, but she finally gave in if I would take lessons. I agreed. (That's how it all started.)

Lessons:
As agreed with Joyce, I took lessons on how to hang glide. My first lesson was in a building in Seattle, WA. The teacher had a hang-glider wing unfolded and hanging from the ceiling. He explained that the pilot was carried during flying by the horizontal bag below the wing, and steering the wing was done by moving the bar on the front and below the wing.

I didn't own a hang glider yet, so I looked in the newspaper for an available used wing for sale. I found a used wing in good shape in eastern WA that included a parachute, all for $500. New wings cost about $3,000.

HOW I BECAME ME

I drove my VW bus to see the used hang glider. The VW bus had been modified to add a roof rack to hook the wing with short lengths of bungee cord should I decide to buy. I examined the wing, and it was perfect, so I bought it and headed home with it fastened to the roof rack.

My second lesson was held in a non-used rock quarry that had a high-to-low distant of about twenty feet. From then on, the classes included using the wing to glide from the high lip to the low floor of the quarry.

I had the parachute repacked by a professional parachute packer. The only thing the instructor found wrong with the parachute was the rubber bands had dried and lost elasticity, and he replaced them all.

High Altitude Flights:
Seven high altitude flights are one of the requirements for the novice. A high altitude flight means the altitude of the landing site is 1,000 feet or more below the altitude of the take-off site. Tiger Mountain and Dog Mountain met that altitude requirement. I flew off both of these sites. After the lessons were over, I moved to the high altitude flights to complete the novice requirements.

FALLING OUT OF NORMAL

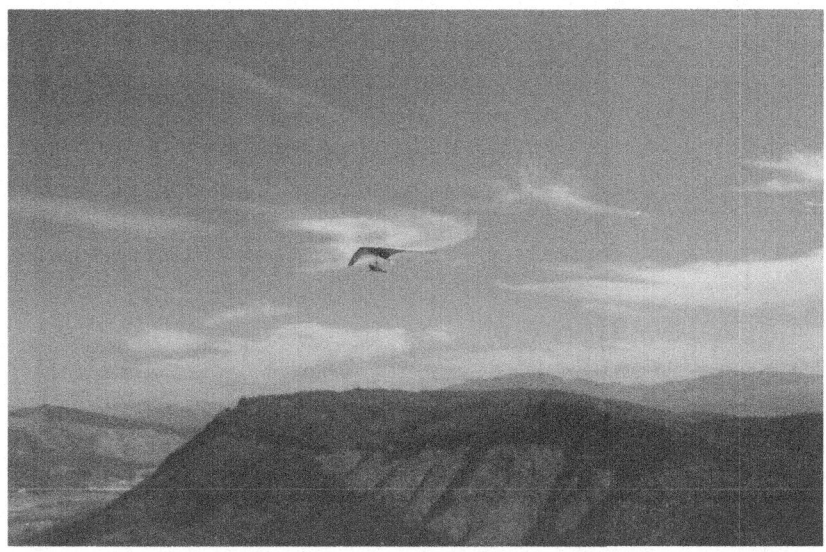

I still remember one of the flights off Dog Mountain. As I approached the landing site, I saw it held two men. As I got lower and lower, the men ran to one side then the other trying to get out of the way. I turned my wing to chase those men. No matter which way they went, I went. At the last moment, I stopped chasing them and made a perfect landing, but boy, was that fun.

Shortly after that, I bought a new motorcycle, so I could use it to drive back up to the top to fetch the VW bus. I would leave the wing at the bottom and ride the motorcycle back to the take-off site.

Plans A & B:
Plan A was for the Pilot to install the two wing nuts which keep the glider from folding.

HOW I BECAME ME

I also saw hang-glider pilots had a Plan B in the case where Plan A failed. With Plan B, an experienced hang glider pilot was supposed to check the wings to be sure that they were ready to fly. The hang glider makers had stopped using the wing nut design because too many pilots were killed by the fall when the glider folded in mid-flight. My hang-glider was an early wing design and still used the wing-nuts.

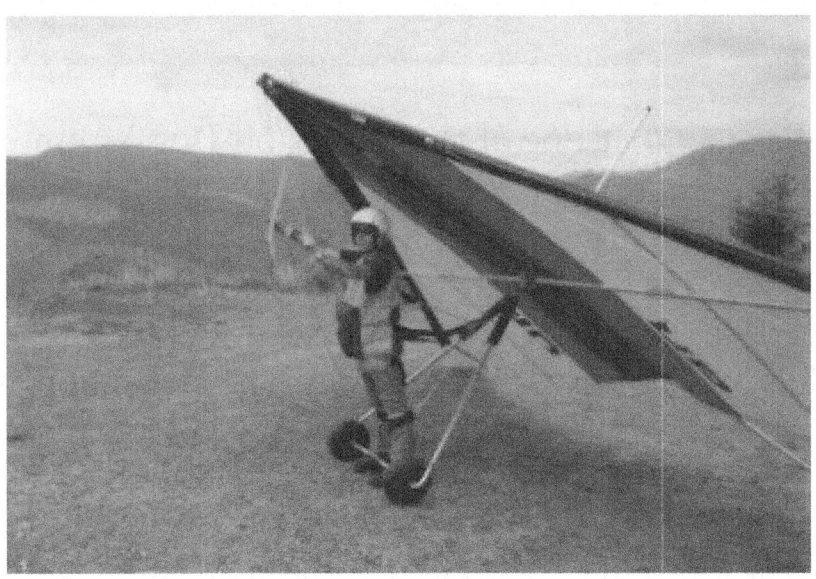

I completed the lessons and practiced on the small hill until I felt ready. I had good high altitude (over 1,000 feet change in altitude "sled rides" no thermals) off Tiger and Dog Mountains, but on my seventh high altitude flight, on 10-20-1984, my life changed. My wing folded in mid-flight. I fell about fifty feet into a tree, then about fifty-five feet through the tree, and hit the ground hard enough to break my fiberglass helmet. I got my first helicopter ride to the hospital. I was later told I never lost consciousness, but I have no memory of the event nor the helicopter ride. The event resulted in five surgeries and two years in a wheelchair because I did not put on two wing nuts. The wing makers do not use wing nuts anymore. Too many pilots forgot to put them on and were killed by the fall. I was told that if you carry them in your mouth, you will remember to put them on, but how do you remember to put them in your mouth? That was after my fall. But, after all is said and done, I did get the chance to read and study a lot because of the injury. In the hospital, I had more than enough time than anything else.

My Injury:
My injury was the result of the failure of both Plans A and B. My wing folded in mid-flight. I was on my seventh high altitude flight, and it was off Dog Mountain. Buying a wheelchair more than exceeded the saving in money I made by purchasing an old wing. I would have saved by buying a new wing. One that used a latter design and would not have folded in mid-flight. I have done a lot of thinking about it and all things considered, the injury was probably the best thing that happened to me during this life. (My soul tells me I am on my 400 plus life, but I don't expect you to believe that, of course. Reincarnation is not even mentioned in the King

HOW I BECAME ME

James Version of the Bible because King James did not believe in reincarnation. He also knew he would lose followers if they knew they could resolve wrong-doing in future lives between God and themselves instead of only through the Catholic church. (BTW: The committee that put together the KJV of the Bible was not about to go against the king, so all that stuff was removed from the edited King James' version of the Bible.)

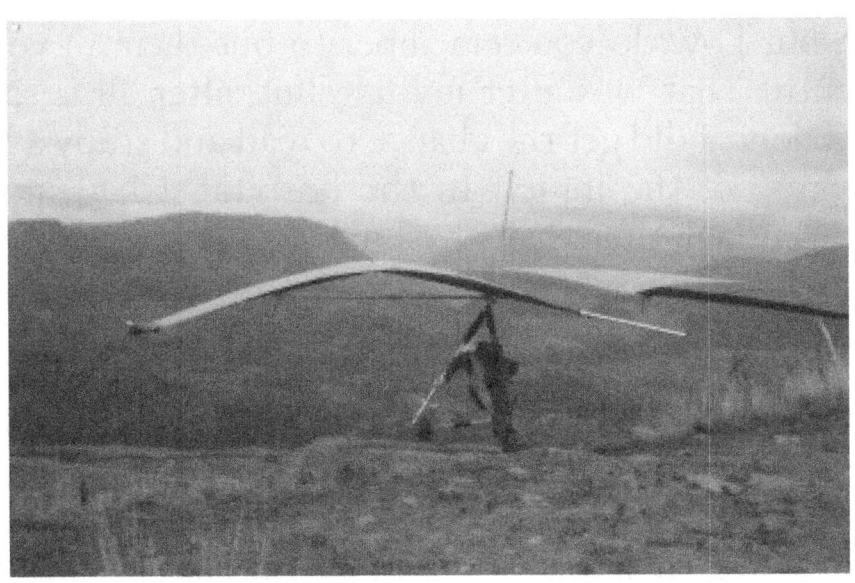

After the wing folded, I fell about fifty feet into a tree, then fifty-five feet through the tree and hit the ground hard enough to break my fiberglass helmet. The others who cared for me determined that no ambulance could get near enough to get me out, so they called for a chopper.

My injuries were pretty severe, but I was at least still alive. They figured they should let the hospital doctors decide how to put me back together; the doctors were trained to do that.

I never deployed the parachute. In retrospect, I concluded that it would have been of no help to me anyway and would have been torn up by the tree.

My left elbow and left eye were visibly damaged by the fall, and they required observation time to determine if the brain had been involved. Actually, the damages went beyond the obvious, but time would tell.

The Hospital:
As far as I know, the chopper took me to the roof of a hospital in Seattle, Washington, where I entered for the care of the hospital staff.

Some of the effects of my fall were visible, but others were not, and I would have to stay in the hospital long enough for the doctors to be sure that they were aware of all the damage.

I was in the hospital for a month and had five surgeries before the doctors were satisfied that they had treated all the damages. Even though my fiberglass helmet was split by the impact with the ground, it had accepted most of the shock and protected my brain. It was a homemade helmet that I made from a motorcycle helmet and painted orange.

The hospital staff was very efficient and did a fine job on me.

At the time of my injury, I was working for Boeing and stationed in a windowless building called "Black Box."

Life in a Wheelchair:
For a long time, I couldn't walk. It seemed like the only solution was to buy a wheelchair. I hated that chair, but with it, I could get around.

Joyce had bought herself a white Trans Am, and everywhere we went, she had to fold the chair, carry it around to the back of the car, and put it into the car's trunk. I got a taste of life in a wheelchair, and I didn't like it. I had turned from a breadwinner into a dependent.

Work on the house had come to a complete stop.

Retirement Years: Enjoying Isolation

"I'm slower than a bullet but faster than a slug."
-Allen

Life:
My life is totally different now, and it probably will be that way until I die. I got to experience many things in this life. Eventually, I learned to walk, slow, but I didn't need a wheelchair anymore.

Changed:
My adopted daughters really earned their keep. They assumed my care. Every night, after I again learned to walk, they would take me for a walk. I eventually moved out and lived with one of the girls.

HOW I BECAME ME

I was in my 83rd year when I started writing this book, and there are things that I did not include, but most of them are the result of my comparison with what I could do when I was younger and stronger. I should be happy for what I can do now, rather than comparing myself to what I could do in some other phase of my life. At least I am alive, and I can walk with a rollator. I have a handicap parking pass and get *first-class parking.*

My daughter acts as my chauffeur and takes me to the store every week as well as anywhere else I want to go. For the last seventeen years, I have lived with Janine. I have my own room, toilet, computer, TV, dog and stuff. I made a lot of mistakes, but I have no regrets. According to my higher self, this was my 420th life. All I can say is: "*It was fun.*"

A Good Event:
Looking back, the fall was probably the best thing that happened to me in this life. It was like being a child again, and as a result of reading numerous books, I came to realize that a lot of the things I had been told were wrong. Honesty and truth are still right, but some beliefs were not right. I became another person. I could see my faults, and they were many. I could not change my past, but I sure could change my now, which would soon become my new past.

FALLING OUT OF NORMAL

Changing Dogs (And Changing Gods):
I always thought of myself as a German Sheppard man, but ever since my big dog, Putt-Putt died (he was half Shar-Pei and half Bulldog, weighed sixty-five pounds, and boy was he strong), I wanted another dog. Putt-Putt was named by my granddaughter after the car in a children's video game. He was replaced by Barklee, who is mostly a black Miniature Poodle and only weighs sixteen pounds. I have had no problem with being pulled over by dog-strength. I say Barklee is mostly a black miniature Poodle because Janine got him at a dog shelter, and neither they nor the vet could figure his exact breed. I didn't much care because I had no intention to show him. I just wanted a dog that was not strong enough to knock me down during a walk. Putt-Putt did that about four times on our morning walks. Another thing I want to write about is that Barklee is the smartest dog I ever saw. He always spends the night with me. As time goes by, I get weaker, and the dog becomes stronger.

(After reading the Bible cover-to-cover 34 times, I finally concluded that since the Bible was written by imperfect men, thus it was untrue in spots and I stopped immersing myself completely in it in 1997. I figured I was an adult by then (67 years old) and could do my own thinking. More than twelve years after my injury, I finally became a non-normal person in 1997 and started learning about Metaphysics and Eastern Philosophy. I got a doctorate in Metaphysics in 2003. In 2009, I was trained in editing and started helping my daughter edit her books.)

Leash Law:
Whereas I use to see a leash only as a restriction on the dog, I now see the leash as a safety device *for* the dog. With it, I can always prevent him from running out in the street in front of a car. I know because of what happened to Putt-Putt. One day the gate was left open, and Putt-Putt got out. Fortunately, the car was going very slowly, but it passed completely over the dog without hitting him with a wheel. The vet said there were no broken bones, and the abrasions would heal. Now I never take Barklee out of the fenced yard except when he is on-leash. The leash has become a safety device. The dog today has his own yard made by my son-in-law.

Attack Mode:
Every morning the alarm was set to go off at seven-thirty, and I would get ready for the day, starting with my morning walk with the dog. It took about fifteen minutes to do everything I had scheduled, then I would be ready to go. The dog was leashed and fastened to the belt around my body. He had a special harness so I could pick him up by the leash without choking him. The harness puts all leash

loads on his chest rather than on his throat. With the dog and Rollator, we would head out. The walk used to be about forty-five minutes long, but I have shortened it to about fifteen minutes. The first obstacle was the gate, which still bears the big warning sign, which was put up while Putt-Putt was alive, and reads, "Beware of Dog." Barklee is little but goes into "attack mode" and barks at people he doesn't know yet. It is funny to see such a little dog go into "attack mode" while wagging his tail. I think it is an instinct-left-over for a small dog that has not been trained out of him yet, but I'm working on it.

Rain:
Metaphysics claims that humans create their own future. I always thought that others created my future, and I didn't even get a vote. So, I set up a situation. I always start the day with a walk, rain or shine. I have "rain gear," even boots to keep my feet dry, but I hate to expend the effort and time to put it on. I decided it would not rain on me today. Every morning I thought, "It will not rain on me today." I have gone most of this year without putting on my rain gear. Often the pavement is wet, but no rain. I heard on TV that so far, this was the wettest year ever recorded.

One of my neighbors ask me what I thought of the snow that fell the other day? It had all melted by the time of my walk, and I didn't even know it had snowed. I can only conclude that my thought has not stopped all rain, just most of it during my walk, or maybe my walk is just during periods of no rain; I don't much care. I am convinced my thoughts make a big difference in my future. I realize that my test was not as comprehensive as it might be, but it was enough to convince me. You decide.

Awe, what the heck, I might as well throw this thought in:

General Description of the Car of the Future:

This whole section is just my prediction of the future. It may not happen, and I don't care if it doesn't. I have no vested interest in the future. I don't want more power or money. Not even God changes the past. The best anyone can do is "observe" what "is" and decide if it should be changed, because it can be, or not. And let me point out: this comes from a man who holds a doctor's degree in Metaphysics. Believe what you want, but I believe we create our own future. Do what you want. It's none of my business what you decide.

The car of the future will be powered by batteries, charged every night via a common plug, four-wheel-drive, and have a plastic frame and body. The car of the future has at least eight reasons for being: 1) low rust (from salt on the road), 2) lower cost (original and repair), 3) lower weight, 4) minimum use of the earth's resources 5) no air pollution, 6) reduced wrecks, 7) much reduced human death and injury and 8) longer average service life. The car will have a range of 100+ miles on all batteries and a full charge, automatically go to two-wheel-drive as batteries are depleted or if commanded. It will continually display the condition of the batteries. (Keep in mind, I'm only in my eighties in age. I don't know everything yet.)

Anti Collision System:
The car of the future will have a surrounding radar system, which will eliminate most collisions. It will be activated whenever the vehicle is in automatic mode. That way, humans entering or exiting the car will not be exposed to radar.

Passenger Heating:
Because the car of the future does not make hot coolant (a high user of energy), hot air may be optional, with the air heated electrically. The car may be made like a motorcycle, where heating of the human being(s) is done with clothing. That system has been used on horses drawn buggies, motorcycles, skies, and horse-drawn sleds, among others. In other words, just put on another sweater

or jacket. Wear a cap, for Pete's sake. I'm a simple fellow, okay? My wife used to call me a cheap scape. (Uh, I mean, my ex-wife.)

Driving:
Driving the car of the future will be different. The vehicle could have three modes of operation: manual, automatic, and parallel parking modes. Moving in and out of a garage could be done in the manual mode. Driving between destinations could be done in automatic. Parallel parking could be done in, what else but the "parallel parking" mode. The future car could check to be sure it is in the manual mode before it can be moved (maybe a green dashboard light). It may be driven out of the garage and onto the street, as long as the car is in manual mode and the maximum speed over-ride has not been commanded. Maximum speed will be automatically set for both forward and reverse (maybe twenty-five MPH, maybe faster, who knows.). The car may be driven in that mode as long as desired. On reaching a "start address," the driver may command automatic mode and type in the "termination address." Once a "start address," the automatic mode, and the "termination address" are commanded, the computer, using Global Positioning System (GPS), determines the best route, and the rest of the trip is "hands-off" and "feet-off." At any time, the driver may grab the steering wheel and take control of the car unless the radar is actively operating to avoid a

collision. In that case, the driver input is ignored. If the driver takes control of the vehicle, it will automatically revert to manual mode, and the brakes will gently be applied to bring the car to the set manual limit speed. This will usually happen at a destination. At any time, the driver may resume control of the vehicle. The automatic part of the trip will be over, and control of the car may be taken back by the driver to find a parking place. Using the radar system for car-spacing in the automatic mode will eliminate most wrecks and human injury. At the moment, 45,000 people a year are killed or injured by car wrecks. Only cars with a radar system will be allowed on the freeways. This alone will be a big reason to buy a new car. The radar system will have a much shorter response time than a human being, so vehicles can travel much closer together (maybe 20 feet apart), allowing the present freeway system to handle more traffic (maybe 10 times as much, or more). The driver might even go to sleep or be drunk and no wreck. An option might be a "parallel parking command" used for parallel parking, also a "hands-off and feet-off" function.

Mode Selection:
In the automatic mode, the system will determine the car's total weight, including car weight, people weight, and cargo weight, and compare round-trip energy to ensure that the vehicle can make it. The driver may always command "one way" if a recharge

is planned en route, like staying overnight. If more than one mode is commanded simultaneously, no mode will be applied.

Call:
The whole call of this proud system is to call a system that doesn't deplete the world's resources nor enhance its poisons. Some of the features might be hard to include. The trip length might require a car that runs on gasoline only or runs on both electricity and gas. The owner might have two cars—one used for short trips, like work, and one for long, like out of state trips.

Millennial Years: Making Peace with Not-Normal

"Just bury me in a nut jar." -Allen

Full Circle:
I am an eighty-eight-year-old (born in 1930) male, raised in Portland, Oregon. I graduated from Jefferson High School in 1948, hold a BS degree in Physics and a Ph.D. in Metaphysics. I was hired in 1951 to work at Boeing. I got married and moved to Seattle, Washington, in 1952, where I worked for Boeing on military products for over thirty-two years. Then I took up hang gliding, which changed my life.

A Brief Recap:
I was a born leader and used the attribute as I matured. My parents had the biggest house in the

neighborhood, and we had a car. We were the only people in the neighborhood who owned a car. All the other kids thought we were rich. Actually, the house was owned by my father's sister.

We lived upstairs for a while, but as the family grew, we move down to the main floor, my father's sister and her husband lived on the top floor, and my father turned the basement into a woodshop.
One day I found my grandfather's snare drum, then took lessons on the snare drum, joined the elementary school orchestra, and finally the Jefferson High School band. Being in the band, I got in free to all the high school games and marched in all the rose festival parades.

Down Time is Normal:
I had spells of depression when I compared what I could do as a younger man to what I could do after the injury. My daughters always seemed to know what to say to get me out of the funk. I no longer use a wheelchair and use nippers to cut my own fingernails, and my daughter trims my toenails. After all, I am not a young man anymore. But the thing that blows me away is controlling the weather.

On Creating:
I talk about creation, and the creation that impresses me the most was changing the weather. I was going for a fifteen-minute walk every morning,

rain or shine. I created a no rain period so I would not get wet during my walk. Now I have a college degree in Physics, so I know what causes rain, but for the last five years, it has only drizzled on me about twice per year and never got me wet. I live in Washington state, and we have a normal rainfall of about thirty-six inches per year. It often rains at night, so the pavement gets wet—but not on me!

I started to think for myself, and that's when I decided that I had been living life by some other human being's rules, and most of their rules were non-productive.

At the root, there are only two basic motives for any action: fear and love. Most people in the world use fear as their basic motive, and they don't even know it. Not only are most of the people living out of fear, but they avoid thinking because it entails effort. The motto of most People is: Let somebody else do the thinking. The book *The Messengers* got me started, and it was soon followed by the trilogy *Conversation With God* for my temporary use. CWG makes a big point of "observation." After that, I turned to Eastern Philosophy for answers. Long talks with my daughter have made life meaningful. She treats me like I'm normal even though she knows I'm not. I have nothing that I once had. I don't even know what became of most of the things I once had. Yet, I have everything I need. Actually, I have more than I need. Now that's an "observation."

I was in my seventies before I realized that life is just a series of events. It is like a movie, which is just a series of still pictures shown in rapid succession. Much of the motivational data I had been given by my parents, my school teachers, and even church ministers were wrong. I'm probably the only minister you'll find that disagrees with organized religion. Your church is inside. Your relationship with your moral compass is private.

Humans are designed to create, but this is hard for me to believe. Every morning I took the dog, Putt-Putt, and then Barklee for a walk. I have been doing this for about ten years and two different dogs. During my walks, I prayed silently for no rain, and I have had rain only about twice a year. It typically rains at night, making the ground wet, but it seldom rains on me.

My job now was to find work-a-rounds. I can do most things, just not as fast as when I was younger. I found that with my work-a-rounds and persistence, I could do most things, just not as fast. One of my favorite sayings is, "I'm slower than a bullet but faster than a slug." This puts me in the category with everyone else. I'm normal, but at the same time, I'm *not normal*.

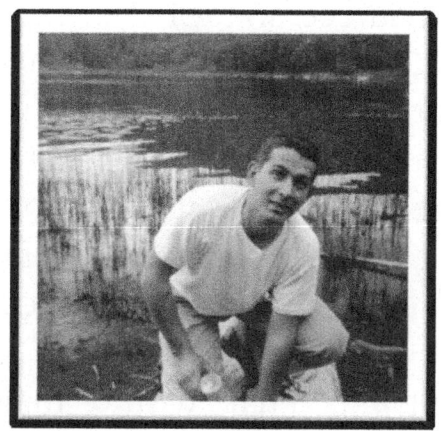

Afterthoughts: Why I Journaled

I advocate for every human to write their life story:

1. Life is a very special thing.
2. We all live in an incredible age.
3. Your life is worth it.
4. It is a way to leave a record of your life.
5. It is a great memory jogger (it is fun).
6. It can be a great learning and teaching tool.
7. I did it because it gave me something to read at the writing group meetings.

HOW I BECAME ME

I think everyone should make some kind of a record of their life: a tape, a disc, a flash drive or a book, whatever you want.

I not only lived, but I did some very unusual things. In any event, never in the history of humans, has technology advanced so rapidly. Many Bible scholars interpreted the Bible to mean that the world would come to an end in the year 2000. Well, that never happened, but something did transpire. Some humans woke up, and I was one of them. When I was growing up, my parents, the schools, the colleges, and churches brainwashed me with what everyone else believed, and I now concluded that they were wrong. That would make at least six billion humans were wrong. I am not trying to convince anyone to believe what I do. I didn't wake up until after my injury. It just goes to show that even old people can wake up.

Another reason for this book is to share what persistence can do. At least that worked for me. Each human is unique, so I can't guarantee that my philosophy will work for you, but I am happy to have the opportunity to share what I believe worked for me.

Allen
PS If I can write a book, you can too!

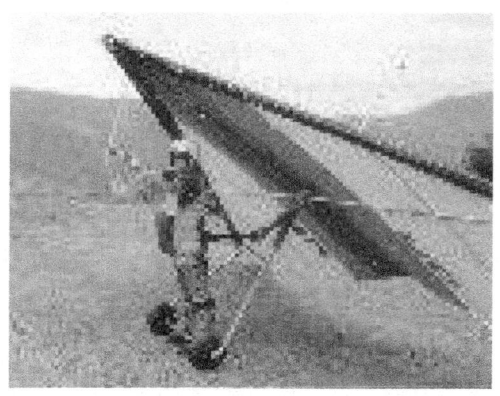

About the Author:
Rev. Dr. Allen Vance, Msc. D.
"The worst thing you can call me is normal."
Allen Vance earned a Doctorate Degree in Metaphysical Science in 2003. Today he most enjoys reading spiritual books, trying different meditation and hypnotherapy techniques, exercising, editing, taking his dog for walks, and solving online puzzles.
Prior to the injury, he earned Master's Degree in Physics with Minors in Math and Philosophy from the University of Portland in 1952. He was hired on at Boeing as a mechanical engineer, and volunteered much time serving as a choir director, church elder, Boy Scout leader, and Sunday School teacher. He now refers to the 100-foot fall in 1984 as the best thing that has happened to him.

HOW I BECAME ME

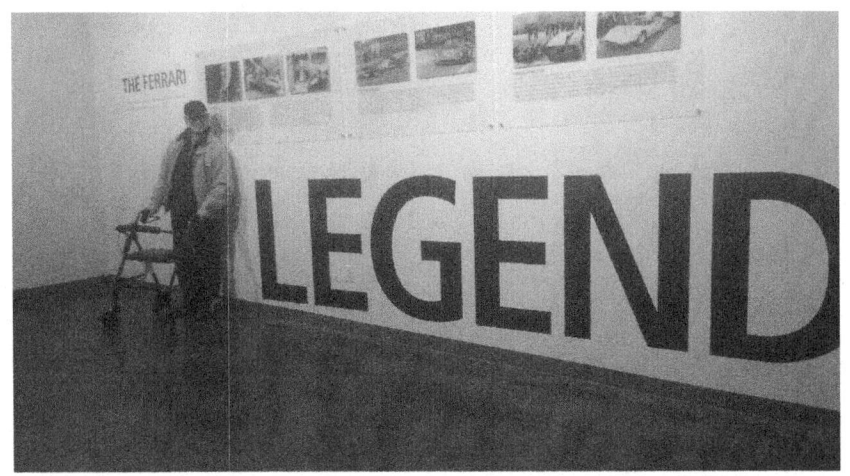

Allen at the LeMay –America's Car Museum

(They called me crazy. But my daughter says maybe that's a great thing. I wouldn't want to be like anyone else. If you liked this book, I'd really appreciate it if you would leave a blurb in the comments section of the online retailer. This helps me feel better about myself. It's been a really tough year. Any words of encouragement would uplift my daughters, too. All of us around the world have gone through so much.)

FALLING OUT OF NORMAL

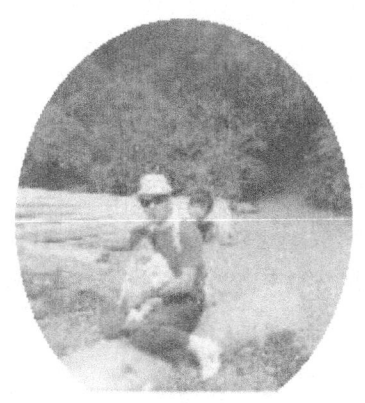

~~~

My story with my twin daughters as told by my daughter, Janine Vance:
Americanized '72: A Generation-X Coming-of-Age (& Identity) Adoption Story

HOW I BECAME ME

Encouragement from Allen
"Don't just *do* something. *Sit there.*"
-Allen Vance
Write for yourself. Write for someone you love.
~~~
Need methods to relax your mind to ease the process of writing and living? This book might help:
Rise from the Dread: A Beginner's Guide to Escape Stress, Worry, and Anxiety.*
This book was edited by me and compiled by my daughter, Janine Vance. It reveals the lifestyle change that I made, which helped me live fully for all these years after my 100-foot hang-gliding fall.

*My daughter included a sample chapter from the paperback book. But you can also read the material in two ebooks if you'd like:
Going Back to Zen & The Power of Isolation.

About
Rise from the Dread

Rise from the Dread sets the stage for individuals who have had life turned upside down, and find it cold, harsh, and abrupt, but do not have time to meditate. For those of us who appreciate the wealth from nature— free stuff that makes life a little bit easier (because nature is healing and can make all the difference in the world), this book is dedicated to you. A tiny shift in focus can change everything.

If you ever find yourself facing surprising or traumatic circumstances and looking for a complementary perspective, I write this to humbly share a tidbit of encouragement. Take whatever resonates with you and discard the rest.

I give my appreciation to all those who have helped with me in life--particularly those individuals who have uplifted and encouraged me at one time or another and can see me for who I am. You know who you are.

As someone who has spent the past twenty years following my curiosity, researching, and writing on a topic that has caused turmoil, the contents of this book represent sources of inspiration, which have fueled my ability to keep going. I hope that at least a few of these techniques will uplift, encourage, and empower you to unite with your greater self.

HOW I BECAME ME
Introduction:
WHEN SHIFT HAPPENS

Have you been too hard on yourself? This book serves as a reminder to trust your inner guidance. You can rely on it! Your instincts are connected to the center of the universe— the bigger picture. Utilize your imagination, play with that energy, and explore that amazing inner self. When you're not in meditation, take life as lightly as possible. Remember, your every thought serves as a prayer to the universe, so create something good.

The exploration into unknown territory can cause anxiety at times, but it can also lead us back to the value and pride of our mysterious ancestral roots. From there, we not only survive, but we can also thrive. Mother Nature requires no belief in her capabilities, nor any worship of any kind. It is up to each individual to decide for themselves their own twist and route.

You are connected to the universal stars. You have the answers to your questions. Just take the time to ask yourself because the people around you need you, shucks, humanity needs you! We need to make this place a more united place— it'll make life easier for all of us! Master each little moment the way you see fit. Doing the most difficult tasks first, bit by bit, suddenly and eventually, with practice, life gets easier. Together, each of us can make the world a sacred space.

I've combined two ebooks *Going Back to Zen* and *The Power of Isolation: How Silence is Golden* in this print book to offer additional tips on setting up a spiritually lucrative meditation practice. I hope that this writing uplifts you, and sets the stage for an easier meditation practice.

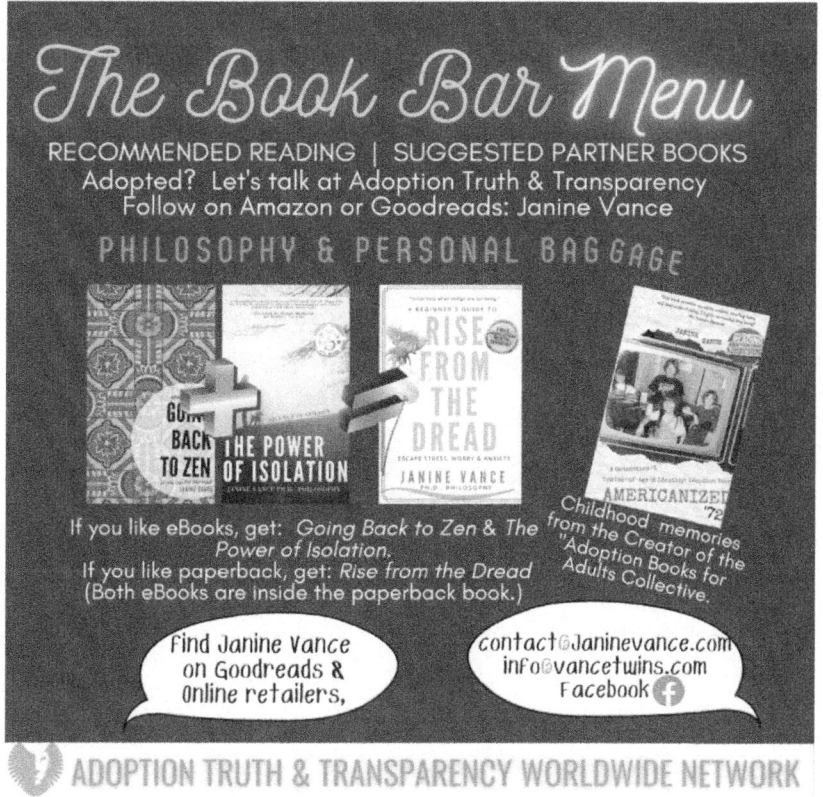

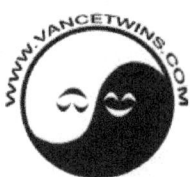

Ever thought about turning your life into a book? Memoirs are a priceless keepsake and serve as a legacy for family. My daughter, Janine, is a bookmaker and offers personalized therapeutic writing sabbaticals for non-writers. My other daughter arranges and manages the sessions:
Email: jenette@vancetwins.com
www.vancetwins.com/

Send the twins a message if you want to order large print editions of their books.

Made in the USA
Coppell, TX
07 August 2021